Jane Garton has been editing and writing for more than twenty years. She started her career as a sub-editor on the *Journal for the Royal Society of Medicine*. She has since worked on numerous publications including *Nursing Times*, *Fitness* and *New Woman*. She was the editor of *Top Santé*, Britain's leading health and beauty magazine from 1993-1997 and is now a freelance editor and writer.

Special thanks to my agent Michael Alcock, my editor, Caroline Oakley, my trusted advisers Vicci Bentley and Dr Brian Piggot, nutritionist Norma Doucet, Dr Rajendra Sharma, medical director at The Hale Clinic, the staff at the Tyringham Clinic who so very kindly helped me with food facts for a healthy diet, Jennifer Blondel, naturopathic consultant at Blackmores, Steve Bedford at the Metropolitan Fitness Club in Fulham and last but not least my friends and family, especially Charles, Vicky, Sarah and my twin sister Annie for their constant support and encouragement.

Also available in Orion paperback

APPLES & PEARS
Gloria Thomas

AROUSING AROMAS
Kay Cooper

EAT SAFELY
Janet Wright

HEALTH SPA AT HOME
Josephine Fairley

JUICE UP YOUR ENERGY LEVELS
Lesley Waters

SPRING CLEAN YOUR SYSTEM

JANE GARTON

ORION

An Orion Paperback
First published in Great Britain in 1998 by
Orion Books Ltd,
Orion House, 5 Upper St Martin's Lane,
London WC2H 9EA

A CIP catalogue record for this book
is available from the British Library.

ISBN: 0 75281 601 2

Printed and bound in Great Britain by
The Guernsey Press Co. Ltd, Guernsey

The author of this book is not a physician, and the ideas,
procedures and suggestions in this book are intended to
supplement, not replace, the medical advice of trained profes-
sionals. Consult your medical practitioner about any condition
that may require diagnosis or medical attention, and before
adopting the suggestions in this book.

CONTENTS

INTRODUCTION

WHY DETOX?

Why spring clean your system? Why detox? Why go for days without the foods you really like? The answer is simple: it will make you feel better in every aspect of your life. You will feel more alive, more alert, more aware and you will look better too. Your hair and skin will start to glow with a new-found radiance.

You may think you're healthy but are you really? Think again for a minute. Do you feel tired 99 per cent of the time? Do you get up in the morning and have to drag yourself to work? When you get there, is every minute an effort? And how about when you get home at night... Is falling asleep in front of the television about all you can manage? You are so used to feeling like this you probably think it's normal, but it's not. It's a sign that your mind and your body are not working as efficiently as they could be, and this is why you need to spring clean your system - to renew your energy and boost your vitality.

It's not surprising that most of us feel below par. From the water we drink to the air we breathe, we are surrounded on all sides by toxins. There's no escaping these harmful substances that irritate our bodies and put undue strains on all our vital organs. What's more, toxicity is a much greater worry than ever before. Industrial chemicals are far stronger, our food is more highly refined and pollution levels are much higher than they were 50 years ago.

Each of us has our own unique self-cleansing and self-healing system designed to absorb and eliminate a certain amount of these toxins. But all too often the amount we inhale and ingest is too great for our bodies to cope with. Our livers, kidneys and immune systems become less efficient under the strain. As the toxins start to circulate around our bodies, blocking channels and robbing our cells of vital nutrients, we start to feel the effects. Headaches, tiredness and irritability are the inevitable result.

But you don't have to live like this, you don't have to put up with this general feeling of malaise. Just as servicing your car will make it run better, so spring cleaning or detoxing your system will help you to perform better at all levels. Removal of waste material - detoxification - is essential for the healthy functioning of your body. There's nothing new about detox - it is a tried and tested method of healing. Hippocrates, the great father of medicine, prescribed it in the short term as one of the most dependable curative and rejuvenating methods known to man, and people have been taking the waters at health spas in Europe for years.

The principle of detox is straightforward - healing through cleansing. If you remove all the toxic ingredients from your diet and replace them with cleansing restorative foods your body will automatically start the healing process. If you limit your intake of food, your body will be able to divert the energy it usually puts into digestion into the important job of getting rid of stored toxins.

How long you devote to a detox programme really depends on your personal circumstances. Weekend and one-day detoxes are great for breaking a cycle of binges, especially after a period of indulgence such as at Christmas. They also provide a quick 'pick me up' if you've been going through a long period of feeling down and lethargic. They give your body time to catch up on its essential housework, while seven-day programmes tackle cleansing at a deeper cellular level.

Once you have experienced the benefits of a detox, there will be no going back. Even a few days is long enough to break old habits. Spring cleaning your system rejuvenates and restores life to your cells and you will realise just how good you can feel. It gives you a new energy and vitality and you will start to see life from a brighter perspective. It will make you realise that a healthy diet, regular exercise, living in the right environment and avoiding stress are the keys to a healthy new you.

CHAPTER 1

Get Toxin Wise

Our bodies have the capacity to clean and heal themselves, but the world in which we live is far from ideal and everyday living puts an enormous strain on this natural bodily process. The fruit and vegetables we eat have been sprayed with pesticides, herbicides or fertilisers; the food we buy in the supermarket has been laced with additives to prolong its shelf life; the water we drink is polluted with chemicals; the air we breathe in the street is full of lead from exhaust fumes and the rooms we live and work in are full of machines emitting fumes, not to mention radiation from VDUs and television screens.

Add to this the pressures of a demanding job, bringing up a family and possibly an unhealthy relationship and it's not surprising that sometimes our bodies say that enough is enough. The human body is amazingly resilient and will put up a strong fight against a barrage of toxins but sooner or later something tends to give and we start to feel below par, or worse, fall ill.

So what can you do? You can't avoid toxins – harmful substances have always existed even within foods whose overall effects are deemed positive – but you can become aware of the major sources of pollution so that you can minimise your exposure to them or protect yourself against their negative effects.

AIR

With every breath you take, you are also inhaling masses of impurities from the air – by-products of 20th-century industry. The atmosphere, especially in built-up urban areas, is laden with airborne pollutants – from cars, cigarettes, industrial plants, gas boilers and office ventilation systems – and each can be a significant threat to our health. Airborne pollutants increase the risk of respiratory diseases, weaken our immune systems and make us more susceptible to cancer and although rural areas are healthier, they don't escape the effects of pollution. Also, scientists are now saying that the health and welfare of the whole planet is under threat as pollution eats away at the earth's protective ozone layer, allowing the delicate balance of forces that control our climate to be upset.

ACTION

- Outdoor pollution is the responsibility of the government but until they decide to bring in tougher health and safety laws and traffic regulations you should do everything you can to reduce or contain it.
- Don't use your car unless you have to. Use public transport, walk or get a lift with a friend.
- Try to avoid walking in areas of heavy traffic and if you do have to venture into heavily polluted areas, try to breathe through your nose – the delicate hairs just inside your nostrils act as a filter, brushing away some of the toxic particles.
- If you ride a bike wear a mask.

SUNLIGHT

We all need some sun to promote the manufacture of vitamin D in our skin but at the same time it pays to be aware of its dangers. The sun is a nuclear power station that emits its energy in the form of ultraviolet (UV) rays. These are filtered out to some extent by the ozone layer that protects the earth, but as this is gradually becoming depleted, the rays are becoming stronger and more dangerous. All types of skin cancer are linked to repeated exposure to UV rays, both A and B, which are also thought to be connected with the production of free radicals.

ACTION

- Never go out in the sun without wearing a sun cream with a protection factor of fifteen or more to filter harmful UVA and UVB rays.
- Don't rely on sunscreen alone. You should limit your time in the sun and always stay in the shade between 11 a.m. and 3 p.m.
- Wear a sun hat or visored cap.
- The antioxidant vitamins A, C and E help protect against free radical damage.

FARMING

Pesticides, fertilisers and herbicides may take some of the hard work out of gardening and farming – they kill weeds, insects and pests as well as foster growth – but they don't just do their job and disappear. They remain in the soil, on the crops, seep into the water and eventually through to our food and drink where they reach us, adding to the toxic build-up. Meat, poultry and dairy farming are not without fault either. Cows and chickens are often given antibiotics to ward off disease and hormones to promote rapid growth which, once within the food chain, are all potentially hazardous to our health. The recent BSE crisis in Britain is also a sharp reminder of what can happen if we interfere with our livestock's natural feeding patterns.

ACTION

- Buy organic produce including meat and poultry whenever possible.
- Always wash fruit and vegetables before eating.

- Remove the outer leaves from leafy vegetables and peel the waxy coating off fruit.
- Avoid buying fruit and vegetables from street market stalls – pollution from car exhaust fumes is too high a risk.
- Thaw all frozen foods completely and make sure that meat is always thoroughly cooked.

FOOD PROCESSING

Most of the food we buy is processed or refined and, although a certain amount of processing is necessary to eliminate harmful bacteria and to give our foods a longer shelf life, it can have extremely toxic and damaging effects on our bodies – especially in the long term. Traditional methods of preserving foods included chilling, salting, smoking

During the refining process, the parts of the food which contain the majority of vitamins and minerals are often discarded.

and drying, but there are now many more including freezing, canning and irradiation, the long-term effects of which are still unknown. All affect the food in some way but some cause more harm than others. During the refining process, the parts of the food which contain the majority of vitamins and minerals are often discarded. For example in the production of white flour, during which the bran, germ and outer husk are thrown away, over half the important B vitamins are also lost. Similarly when food is canned, vitamin C and many of the B vitamins are lost. Salt is also added, which can upset the delicate sodium/potassium balance in our bodies. Food additives – chemicals added to give colour, sweetness or simply to preserve or stabilise food – are another potential nightmare but it is still too early for their long-term effects to be established. Irradiation, a relatively new process developed to extend the shelf life of foods is the latest worry. High energy rays are used to disrupt DNA and to kill the bacteria responsible for food going off. Irradiation also causes chemical changes in foods that may or may not be harmful – it is still too early to say.

ACTION

- Replace processed and packaged foods with fresh natural produce wherever possible.
- If you do buy processed foods read the labels carefully and be aware of E additives.
- If you are concerned about irradiation, join consumer groups that are calling for more research into its effects, for restrictions on its use and for full disclosure on labels.
- Get in touch with FLAG (the Food Labelling Agenda) a pressure group set up by the Guild of Health Writers and the Guild of Food Writers which is campaigning for better labelling of our foods so that the consumer knows exactly what ingredients they contain (see p.120).

BEWARE E NUMBERS

Many manufacturers are now using the technical name instead of the E number to avoid having to disclose some additives on the label. Watch out for the following:
- E951 (aspartame) A sweetener, found in snacks, concentrated fruit juices, sweets and fizzy drinks, which can bring on headaches
- E129 (allura red AC) A food colouring, used in snacks, sauces, preserves and soups, which can aggravate asthma or hay fever symptoms
- E220 (sulphur dioxide) A preservative in many foods, including dried fruit, burgers and biscuits, which reduces the absorption of essential vitamins and minerals
- E330 (citric acid) Used for flavouring, too much of which can cause tooth decay and mouth irritation
- E418 (gellan gum) A thickening agent, used in soups and sauces, which can cause diarrhoea if taken in high doses.

OFFICES

Despite their high-tech appearance, modern office blocks are a major source of toxins. As more and more buildings are being built with sealed windows, and open plan offices remain lit by fluorescent light, furnished synthetically and equipped with inefficient heating and ventilation systems, so a growing number of people are starting to suffer from what they call in America poor IAQ (indoor air quality). An unhealthy cocktail of trapped bugs is being steadily released into the atmosphere and the result is a whole range of irritations for the skin, eyes, nose and throat.

ACTION

- If possible, open the windows whenever you can and try to get out into the fresh air during your lunch hour.
- Insist that the office is a non-smoking zone.
- Make sure air-conditioning vents and heating systems are working properly and are uncovered. Both should be serviced at regular intervals.
- Buy an ioniser from your local electrical supplier. These help to rid the atmosphere of a build-up of undesirable positive ions and to recharge the negative ions, sometimes known as 'air vitamins', found in largest numbers by the sea and on mountains.
- Increase humidity levels, especially if you work on a computer (the heat of which can dry the air, causing and aggravating skin problems).
- Surround yourself with pollution-hungry plants. Those that are said to reduce pollution in the atmosphere include Cereus Peruvianus (Mexican cactus) and Chlorophytumelatum (the familiar spider plant).

WATER

Pure water contains no toxins, but during the past fifty years our drinking water has become more and more contaminated. Most comes from a main supply and contains additives which, although added to clean up our water, have the potential to damage our health. Drinking tap water containing aluminium, often added during the purification process to remove particles which

> *Only half of the nitrogen put on fields as fertiliser is taken up by plants.*

colour water brown, has been linked to Alzheimer's disease. Only half of the nitrogen put on fields as fertiliser is taken up by plants. The rest drifts down into our water supplies and high levels of nitrates have been found to have and adverse effect on health. Chlorine is added to water to kill bacteria, but it reacts with peat and other organic material that are found in water to form a group of chemicals which have been linked with cancer. Lead from old piping is another hazard. It can seep out of the pipes into the water flowing through them and is particularly toxic to children and unborn babies. Lead has also been shown to stunt growth and to damage the brain and nervous system.

ACTION

- Find out exactly what's in your water from your water supplier (listed under water in *Yellow Pages*). They should also be able to tell you how your water compares with the water supply (water-quality) regulations.
- If you do drink tap water, always run it for a couple of minutes before drinking to make sure it's as fresh as it can be, and don't drink water from the hot tap. Hot water is usually stored in a plastic or metal tank and as water is a natural corrosive the surrounding material may well have seeped into it.
- Drink bottled water. As there are almost as many different types as there are brands it is worth reading and understanding the labels, so you know what you are buying. 'Natural mineral water' means that the water has come from a specified underground source, that it has satisfied micro biological criteria and is free of harmful bacteria. A wide

range of waters are described as 'Spring', and 'Natural' water. These may be drawn from any source and may be processed to remove harmful bacteria or chemicals. If the label reads 'Table' or just 'Purified' it may well have come straight from the mains tap having been first treated and disinfected according to a set of regulations. It may also have been filtered and contain mineral salts.

It's up to you to shop around, to find a brand you like and to stick to it. Remember that bottled water like any other water goes off after a while so throw away unfinished bottles after a day or two. Leaving bottles in the sun should also be avoided – as the plastic of the bottle starts to warm up it can taint the water.

Filter water. The cost of drinking bottled water on a daily basis can soon add up and filtering your own water is a cheaper option. Special active carbon filters, which work by removing the chemicals as they pass through them, can be plumbed in under the kitchen sink or attached to the end of the kitchen tap. The least expensive option is a jug filter. A plastic lid containing an active carbon filter fits on top of the jug and filters the water as it is poured through. These can be very effective but you must remember to wash the jug and filter regularly, and to change the filter at least once a month.

STRESS

Life in the Nineties is busy. We are all under an enormous pressure to work hard, to play hard, to be high achievers, but we often fail to recognise the enormous toll this is taking on our bodies. Physically we react by producing huge amounts of adrenaline in response to stressful situations. All our energy is diverted into coping with the stress and is diverted away from the important digestive processes – we don't get the essential nutrients from our food and our bodies won't have done the necessary repair and maintenance work.

WHAT HAPPENS WHEN STRESS STRIKES

Stressful situations trigger a chain of biochemical and physical reactions which correspond to what is known as the stress curve. This consists of three main stages: alarm, overstress and exhaustion. The alarm phase happens when you are faced with a challenge – whether it's a child running out in front of your car, your partner being unfaithful, or being given a deadline at work – and its purpose is to prepare you for action. The stress hormones, adrenaline, non-adrenaline and cortisol flood into the bloodstream and mobilise energy stores, creating a feeling of alertness. Your physical and mental abilities become sharper and you tend to block out everything except the challenge. As long as you have the chance to wind down or defuse the tension with some type of exercise as soon as the stressful situation has subsided, there are no long-lasting effects on the body.

If, however, you are constantly in a state of stress, your body remains in a state of arousal and its energy stores become depleted as you struggle to meet the persistent demands. What's more the stress hormones start to build up, adding to the toxicity in your body. This is known as the overstressed phase when you gradually become less able to cope mentally and physically. Depression and lethargy are common symptoms. Now is the time to stop and take action before you slip into the third phase which is exhaustion.

If the stress continues and your body doesn't get the chance to recover then exhaustion sets in.

If the stress continues and your body doesn't get the chance to recover then exhaustion sets in. At this stage you are likely to start feeling ill. Indigestion, persistent diarrhoea and eating disorders are clear signs that you could be suffering from toxic stress.

ACTION

- Try to respond rather than react to stressful situations by making self-help techniques such as yoga, meditation and deep relaxation exercises part of your daily life (see p. 84).
- In moments of stress taking a few deep breaths can help: breathe in through your nose for two to three seconds, pause for a second, then breathe out to a count of seven or eight. Repeat until the anxiety passes.
- Take regular exercise and get plenty of rest and sleep (see p106).

YOUR HOME

Even the cleanest home can be a potential source of toxic poisoning. Old paint, asbestos tiles, damp-proof treatments, roof insulation all contain harmful chemicals which you can do little about, but a few simple steps can vastly improve your indoor environment.

ACTION

- Avoid synthetic wall-to-wall carpeting. Instead, choose natural fibres or wool.
- Go for wood furnishings and avoid anything plastic.
- Open the windows and make sure there's always plenty of fresh air circulating.
- Get gas fires and boilers checked regularly for leaking carbon monoxide fumes and make sure you have adequate ventilation. You can also buy carbon monoxide detectors which should be placed near the fire or boiler.
- Install ionisers.
- Most paints are perfectly safe but if you are prone to allergies or headaches go for brands that are water based or solvent free.
- Use non-toxic household products.

FREE RADICALS

Free radicals are unstable oxygen atoms that have unpaired electrons spinning around them. They are the natural by-product of oxidation – the process by which the body converts oxygen into energy – and are needed in small amounts by the body to kill off harmful bacteria. However, they can also be triggered by pollutants such as cigarette smoke, car exhaust fumes, and UV radiation from the sun. If left unchecked, they can age cells and even destroy them by damaging their structure and DNA.

ACTION

- Try to avoid factors which trigger free radicals, such as cigarette smoke, pollution and overexposure to the sun.
- Antioxidants protect cells from free radical damage so make sure you eat plenty of foods rich in antioxidants. These include the all-important nutrients beta carotene, vitamins C and E.

Best sources of beta carotene
Carrots, broccoli, tomatoes, spinach, cantaloupe melon, mango and apricots.

Best sources of vitamin C
Oranges, blackcurrants, strawberries, green peppers, kale, Brussels sprouts and tomatoes.

Best sources of vitamin E
Avocado, sunflower seeds, sunflower oil, whole grains and soya beans.

CHAPTER 2

How The Body Detoxes

D espite the toxic world in which we live, our bodies are amazingly resourceful and don't just passively absorb harmful substances. We are all born with our own unique self-cleansing system that is constantly on the look out for foreign bodies. For example, it spurs into action as soon as food enters our mouth, filtering out good ingredients from bad, making sure we extract the best nutrients so essential for cell repair, and expelling any toxic substances as well as it can.

Our bodies deal with toxins by either neutralising, transforming or getting rid of them. The liver helps transform toxic substances into harmless ones, the intestines break down protein, carbohydrates and fats, while the kidneys filter waste from the bloodstream. We also sweat out toxins through the skin, and the lymph system clears debris from the blood. Last but not least comes the immune system, which has the important job of fighting bacteria and other foreign invaders.

We are all born with our own unique self-cleansing system

How well this self-cleansing process works depends on your genes, the general state of your health and the extent of your toxic overload. For many of us too much junk food, general pollution and everyday stress mean that our eliminative functions have become impaired. We have taken in more toxins than we can get rid of. Our bodies are finding it difficult to cope and are storing them in our tissues where they are standing in the way of our general well-being and, for all we know, sowing the seeds of disease. It's not all bad news, though. A little spring cleaning could be all that's needed to start to reverse this toxic trend and set the stored poisons free. The first step is to take a look at the body's self-cleaning mechanisms and the vital role of the eliminative organs. If you help them they will help you. As you will see there are many ways in which the body can get rid of toxins, but you can greatly aid this process by making sure the exit path is as clear as possible.

THE IMMUNE SYSTEM

Unlike other systems in the body, the immune system is not confined to one area – it works through many organs and tissues and forms the body's first line of defence, protecting it against foreign intruders. Think of it as a huge army of killer cells whose job it is to protect you against possible invasion by bacteria, viruses and harmful toxins. As soon as it senses that something is a threat to your well-being it steps in, putting up an immediate barrier to prevent the foreign body penetrating any further. The mucous membrane in your mouth, nose and vagina, the small hairs in your nose and ears that stop germs entering, the tears in your eyes – these are all part of the immune system's first line of defence. For example, when your eyes start to water in a smoky room it is a sign that your immune system is reacting with a show of tears to wash away the irritating toxin. If an invader does manage to get through the barrier, the immune system brings out its legion of killer white cells which trigger the production of antibodies and other agents designed to stop the infection in its track.

Sadly, many aspects of modern life such as overuse of antibiotics, smoking, lack of exercise, a fast-food diet and too much alcohol can weaken the immune system. The result is that it is no longer strong enough to put up a good fight against the

> *Overuse of antibiotics, smoking, lack of exercise, a fast-food diet and too much alcohol can weaken the immune system.*

enemy and you start to feel below par, or to suffer constant colds and infections. If this happens recognise it as a signal that your immune system needs support in its defensive role. The first thing to do is to look at your diet. Make sure you are eating enough fruit and vegetables, especially carrots which are rich in beta carotene – known to help strengthen immune barriers. Vitamin C is also essential to a healthy immune system which is why fruit is so important – oranges, blackcurrants and strawberries are all good sources. Another immune booster is regular daily exercise. Walking raises levels of natural killer cells, while research shows that practising less strenuous forms of exercise such as t'ai chi can be beneficial. The gentle flowing movements are said to be particularly effective against anxiety and stress, both factors that can depress the immune system.

THE LIVER

This is not only your biggest organ, it's also the most complex. It is the body's main processing plant, performing over 500 different functions. First and foremost, though, it is a massive filter, the major filter of the bloodstream. It screens every drop of blood entering it and any toxins are immediately set upon by liver cells and deactivated.

The liver regulates blood sugar levels by removing any glucose that is not needed by the body's cells and storing it as glycogen; it processes and stores nutrients such as vitamins A, B, D, E and K; it absorbs alcohol, drugs and other toxins from the blood and alters their chemical structure, to make them soluble so that they can then be disposed of; and it manufactures bile, a greenish brown alkaline fluid that aids the absorption of fats and carries away waste products for excretion. Its smooth functioning is vital to the body's self-cleansing process but all too often, mostly through eating the wrong foods, we overload it and greatly weaken its ability to detoxify. As a result substances get stored in the liver and in fat cells throughout our body and their bad influence on our good health starts to show. Tiredness, lethargy and an inability to concentrate are just some of the more common symptoms. The liver, however, is incredibly resilient and with some extra care and attention we can help it to do its job more efficiently.

Most of our livers need a break. Even if you have constantly overloaded yours with an excess of rich foods, too much alcohol not to mention nicotine, endless cups of coffee and other pollutants it's not too late to remedy the situation. The liver has an amazing power to regenerate itself and giving it some time off via a gentle cleansing programme can get the process going. Dandelion root tea is said to be a good liver tonic and many people believe taking extracts of the seeds of milk thistle (Silybum marianum) stimulates regeneration of liver cells, helping to protect them from toxic injury. You should be able to find it in your local healthfood store where it is usually sold under the names milk thistle, silybum or silymarin (see p. 42).

THE KIDNEYS

Considering their size – 150g heavy and 10-15cm long – the kidneys are very powerful. Their main job is to filter and purify the bloodstream which they do all day long, converting waste into urine. They also salvage and reabsorb valuable nutrients which can be recycled for future use by the body. As with your liver, an unhealthy diet, overuse of drugs or overexposure to toxins can place a great strain on this clever filter system. Smoking cuts down blood flow to the kidneys and a high protein diet is said to put undue stress on these organs. The two most important things you can do to protect your kidneys are to drink lots of water to help flush toxins out and to cut down your intake of protein which basically means eating less meat and dairy products. Try also to avoid eating too much spinach, rhubarb and Swiss chard, which can lead to a build-up of oxalic acid crystals in the kidneys.

THE LUNGS

You may not realise it but your lungs play a major role in the self-cleansing process so it pays to keep them in good shape. Today's environment makes proper breathing techniques more important than they have ever been. Most of the air you inhale is polluted with smoke and chemicals, both of which can damage your lung tissues, causing a secretion of mucous which can reduce the transfer of oxygen into, and carbon dioxide out of, your blood stream.

The main function of breathing is to supply cells via the bloodstream with the necessary oxygen they need to live and to remove carbon dioxide (the waste product of the energy produced by cells) back into the air. Although breathing is instinctive, most of us

Although breathing is instinctive most of us would feel a lot better if we spent some time improving our technique.

would feel a lot better if we spent some time improving our technique. Since the healthy working of all your body systems depends on receiving oxygen and getting rid of carbon dioxide you should aim to move as much air in and out of your lungs as you can. Paying more attention to how you breathe and practising a few simple exercises can make all the difference to how you feel.

BREATHE ON

1 Wear loose comfortable clothes. Lie on your back on the floor or your bed and place both hands on the lower edges of your ribs. Your finger tips should be touching.
2 Breathe in through your nostrils, feel your diaphragm pulling

out and down, your stomach rising and your ribs expanding upwards and outwards. Hold your breath for a few seconds.

3 Breathe out smoothly, making sure you exhale all the air you took in. Allow your ribs to collapse down and in, and your stomach to lower.

4 Repeat three to four times, then relax. Breathe naturally before starting the sequence again.

• If you feel dizzy or faint, relax and breathe normally for a few minutes. The sensation is due to your brain receiving larger amounts of oxygen than it is used to and it will soon pass.

THE SKIN

Your skin is an important eliminative organ. Every pore is an escape route for waste material and when other routes are functioning below par your skin often steps in on a mercy mission. This is why your skin will often break out in spots and blemishes if you are run down or have been overindulging. The best way to give your skin a helping hand in its detoxifying role is to make sure your circulation is as good as it could be and your pores are wide open to allow toxins to escape. External stimulation via brushing and washing (see p. 70) does wonders for your circulation, bringing toxins to the skin's surface and cleaning out the pores. Similarly saunas, steam baths and, at home, hot baths laced with Epsom salts or therapeutic essential oils can be extremely beneficial.

Saunas, steam baths and, at home, hot baths laced with Epsom salts or therapeutic essential oils can be extremely beneficial.

THE DIGESTIVE SYSTEM

You are what you eat, so the saying goes, and the job of converting what you eat into what you are lies with the digestive system. As food travels from the mouth to the bowel, every inch of the intestines is designed for its own particular food-processing role so that the maximum goodness can be extracted and the residue removed from everything that passes your lips. If your stomach and intestines are working well and are processing the food you eat as they should, your body will be absorbing nutrients efficiently and you will feel fit and healthy.

We all have bacteria, known as intestinal flora, living in our gut which help this process, promoting healthy digestion and producing important nutrients such as vitamin K. Although some of the bacteria are potentially harmful, most are not and in a healthy body the good and the bad live together in harmony. Some such as the friendly bacteria Bifido-bacteria and lactobacilus acidophilus are amazing agents of detoxification. They help break down your food, keep the bowel contents moving along and hold some of the less friendly inhabitants of your gut such as candida albicans (thrush) at bay.

Sometimes, however, problems can arise. A bad diet, stress or the overuse of antibiotics can upset this delicate balance. If the bad bacteria become too dominant they can hinder the smooth working of the digestive process. When this occurs the growth of the good bacteria becomes restricted and they can no longer carry out their important protective function and yeasts and bacteria such as thrush start to thrive. Food also remains undigested in the gut and eventually the undigested mass can start to penetrate the intestinal walls and get into the bloodstream, a situation known as leaky gut syndrome.

While many substances, such as pesticides, food additives and alcohol are toxins in their own right, ordinary foods can become toxic if they're not digested or absorbed properly. So before you start any cleansing or detox programme it is important to make sure your gut is healthy. This is one reason why a pre-detox diet (see p. 53) is so important. Supplementing the diet with digestive enzymes can also help. Acidophilus taken in capsule form can help to restore a healthy balance of intestinal flora, ginkgo biloba and antioxidants such as vitamins A and C can help reduce damage, while zinc and glucosamine can help to heal the gut.

It is not difficult to tell when your digestive system is not working as it should. Waves of nausea, feeling bloated, recurring thrush, and frequent bouts of indigestion are all signs.

THE LYMPH

Many of the body's own toxins get drained away through your lymphatic system. In fact, waste drainage is so important to healthy cell functioning that your lymph system is three or four times larger than your bloodstream. What we tend to forget, though, is that it is only designed to remove cell waste. When the blood is also dumping toxins from the intestinal tract into the lymph system via the overloaded liver the lymph system tends to become overloaded too.

So how does it work? While nutrients and oxygen are transported to the cells via the blood, the lymph, a milky white liquid, removes any cellular waste. The system is made up of a vast network of ducts and channels broken up by nodes in the groin, under the arm and in the neck. Its function is to transport the waste to the nearest node where it is filtered to remove impurities then returned to the heart and pumped back into the bloodstream.

While your bloodstream has your body's pump, the heart, to keep it moving, the lymphatic system has no such luck. It relies totally on the actions of your muscles to keep it moving, which is why lymphatic massage and regular exercise can be so instrumental in preventing a build up of toxic wastes in your body (see p. 75).

(see p. 75)

> *Regular exercise and lymphatic massage can be so instrumental in preventing a build up of toxic wastes*

TAKE STOCK

As with all mechanisms, the body's self-cleansing system will work more efficiently if you feed it the right fuel – a balanced diet with the right amount of carbohydrates, protein, fat, vitamins and minerals will give us a much better chance of feeling full of energy and living life at the optimum. But this is where most of us fall down. Our diets are low in fibre, full of highly refined carbohydrates, stimulants, saturated fat, salt, additives, sugar and preservatives. As a result we suffer indigestion, bloating, cramps, constipation, skin impurities and other allergic reactions which are all the result of poor elimination. These are all obvious signs that it is time to take stock. In the short term you can do this by giving your digestive systems a well-earned rest, and in the long term by changing your diet and re-evaluating certain other aspects of your lifestyle such as exercise routines, stress levels, drinking and smoking habits, and by reducing your exposure to outdoor pollution (see p. 92).

(see p. 92)

ARE YOU AS HEALTHY AS YOU THINK YOU ARE?

However healthy you think you are, most of us would benefit from following a gentle cleansing programme if only to dust away the cobwebs. Toxins lurk in unexpected places. Studying and answering yes or no to the following questions should help you to establish if your lifestyle really is as healthy as you think.

Diet

Do you take sugar?
Do you eat white bread and pasta?
Do you regularly eat fast foods such as pizzas and hamburgers?
Do you eat red meat?
Do you use sauces such as ketchup?
Do you eat crisps?

Stimulants

Do you smoke?
Do you drink more than the safe limit of alcohol a day?
Do you drink more than two or three cups of coffee or tea a day?
Do you take medication on a regular basis?
Do you drink canned drinks?

Daily Lifestyle

Do you work in an office?
Do you use a photocopier regularly?
Do you use a mobile phone?
Do you watch a lot of television or work in front of a computer screen?
Do you drive a car?
Do you live in a city?
Do you use household cleaning products?

Symptoms

Do you feel tired a lot of the time?
Are you constipated?
Do you suffer from a dry mouth?
Do you have difficulties in sleeping?
Do you get frequent headaches?
Is your skin or hair dry or coarse?
Do you crave sweet foods?
Are you irritable and defensive?
Do you get indigestion or feel bloated?
Do you suffer mood swings?

HOW DO YOU RATE?

The more yes's you scored the more toxic you are. If you scored four or more in each of the sections your toxic levels are on the high side and it is time for you to look at your diet and lifestyle, which on all counts is far from healthy. You are eating the wrong foods, relying on too many stimulants, living in an unhealthy environment and possibly exposing yourself to too many stressful situations. Now is the time to take stock of yourself physically and mentally.

Giving your system a thorough clean and rest will rejuvenate and refresh you.

Giving your system a thorough clean and rest will rejuvenate and refresh you. You will emerge feeling much stronger and with a more positive outlook on life.

CHAPTER 3

Detox Foods

A poor diet can upset the balance of your natural body functions, disrupting your body chemistry and your blood sugar levels, depleting your energy reserves, making you feel tired and below par, ageing you faster and putting you on the road to illness and disease. You can reverse this situation by giving your system a gentle detox and by paying more attention to what you do and don't eat.

Anything that supports your elimination process can be said to help you detoxify. Just drinking an extra litre of water a day will help you to get rid of toxins, while eating more fruit and vegetables will mean less congestion in your digestive system, enabling food to pass through your body faster. Replacing wheat, animal and dairy products, alcohol, coffee, tea and sugar with more natural alternatives, even for just a few days, can make all the difference.

PLANT POWER

To get the most out of life and a full quota of energy you need to eat high-energy food which is why fruit and vegetables are so important. They are the richest source of live nutrients. Packed with essential vitamins, minerals, amino acids and enzymes, they have got great cleansing properties as well. And it is this ability to clean and revitalise which makes them a must on any detox programme. Some are better at it than others, with most fruit being higher up the cleaning scales than vegetables. Fruits act more as cleansers of the system, while vegetables maintain, repair and build up the cells and tissues of the body. Fruit and vegetables are also full of antioxidants – weapons much needed by the body for fighting off free-radicals. These are the unstable molecules generated by toxins,

> *Fruits act more as cleansers of the system, while vegetables maintain, repair and build up the cells and tissues of our body.*

which if left unchecked can cause great damage to our cells.

All fruits contain a certain amount of fruit acid which is the key to their cleansing power. For example, tartaric acid, found in grapes and pineapples, can stop the growth of harmful moulds and bacteria, while malic acid found in apples, apricots, lemon, peaches, prunes, plums and many other fruits, is a natural anti-septic and helps to cleanse the liver, kidneys, intestines and stomach. Lemons are full of citric acid which probably has the strongest cleansing action of all – in fact it is so strong that lemons often don't appear on gentler detox diets. Other fruits such as oranges and apples also contain pectin which can absorb toxins from the digestive tract.

Fruit and vegetables are also rich in amino acids which are essential for digesting and absorbing food. Once digested they have a strong alkaline effect on the body, which for most of us who live on an over-acid diet of animal protein, sugar, bread and cereals, is a bonus. Like all living things our bodies have a subtle Ph balance between acid and alkaline, with the ideal alkaline level being slightly higher than the acid. Eating plenty of fruit and vegetables helps to restore and maintain this balance.

BEST FRUITS

Apples are rich in fibre and contain pectin, tannic and malic acid, which all help to clean out the intestines and regulate the bowel. They are also rich in beta carotene and are a good source of calcium, while their potassium and phosphorus content helps to flush out the liver and kidneys. The pips contain vitamin E, so don't leave them out if juicing.

Apricots are a good source of vitamin C, beta carotene, potassium and calcium and can help constipation. Remember that dried apricots lose much of their goodness in the drying process.

Grapes, especially the black varieties, contain tannin which helps to speed up the metabolism. They have a high magnesium content, which makes them excellent internal cleansers for the liver, kidneys and other eliminative organs. For these reasons they are the number one fruits in many detox programmes.

Grapefruit have a high level of pectin and fibre, both of which can help digestive problems. The pectin is found in the white pith so don't be too fussy when peeling.

Papayas are well known for their digestive properties. They contain papain, a powerful enzyme which helps the digestion of protein. They can also help to restore a healthy balance of good bacteria after a course of antibiotics. Papayas combine well with pineapples which are also rich in digestive enzymes. Try to buy them when green and unripe as they tend to have more active papain than when ripe.

Pears are high in fibre and pectin and are often included in cleansing programmes for their mild diuretic and laxative effects.

Pineapples contain an important enzyme, bromelain, which helps to break down protein and dissolve excess mucous. They can neutralise excess acidity in the stomach so are good for balancing the body's acid/alkaline levels.

Melons, especially watermelons, have a high water content which makes them an excellent diuretic, and they are also good for cleansing the kidneys. Most of the nutrients are to be found in the flesh nearest the skin so take care when peeling. They should also be eaten by themselves as they pass through the system at a much faster rate than other fruits.

Bananas are high in fibre and pectin, which bind with toxins, helping to remove them from the system, but they do have a high starch content which can make them difficult to digest unless they are eaten when very ripe.

BEST VEGETABLES

Asparagus is a good source of potassium, sodium, manganese and iron. It is more than ninety per cent water and has strong cleansing properties, especially for the kidneys and bladder. It should be eaten raw as when cooked it can irritate the kidneys.

Beetroot juice is one of the most powerful cleansers and is often known as a liver tonic. Its high vitamin A content makes it good for the digestive and lymphatic systems, and for helping the elimination of toxins. The dark green tops which are rich in beta carotene and chlorophyll can be juiced as well.

Cabbage is a good source of vitamins A, C and E, and is rich in calcium, potassium, sulphur, phosphorus, chlorine and iodine. The combination of sulphur and chlorine has a cleansing action on the stomach and intestines.

Carrots also high in the vitamins A, C and E, and have many health-giving qualities, including the ability to soothe and strengthen the intestinal walls. They can also have a cleansing and restorative effect on the liver.

Celery is said by some to help to purify the blood and lymph, and a combination of celery and apple is said to clear away excess carbon dioxide from the body – good news if you live in a polluted area.

Cucumber is easy to digest and its high water content makes it a powerful diuretic. It is also said to have a cleansing effect on the bowels and the skin.

Fennel is rich in sodium, potassium and iron and besides, being a diuretic, it is said to be good for stimulating the lymph and the digestive process.

Lettuce is rich in calcium, magnesium, iron, potassium, vitamins A and E and chlorophyll, and is one of the most nourishing foods for the cells and tissues. The outer leaves are the most valuable as these contain most of the vital nutrients.

- You should avoid tomatoes and spinach when detoxing as they contain large amounts of oxalic acid which can irritate the gut.

GO RAW

To get the maximum nutritional benefit out of fruit and vegetables it is better to eat them raw than cooked. They are easier and quicker to digest uncooked and many of the valuable vitamins, minerals and enzymes tend to get lost in the cooking process anyway. Health guru Leslie Kenton stresses the importance of eating raw food because it contains what she calls 'structural information', which means the food is living, that its cells are alive and contain vital enzymes and minute electrical charges which are then passed on to us. Kenton believes that fifty to seventy-five per cent of food should be eaten raw for this reason.

Fruit can be digested at a much faster rate than most other foods so it is better to eat them separately or at least half an hour before a meal. If eaten as part of a meal they can remain in the stomach for too long and start to putrefy.

JUICE IT

A healthy alternative to raw fruit and vegetables is to juice them down to a healthy drink. Fresh fruit and vegetable juices, whether drunk as part of a detox programme or by themselves on a one-day detox (see p. 67) have been shown to have remarkable healing and cleansing powers. Drinking nothing but fruit or vegetable juice is one of the best ways to start breaking down a build-up of toxins at cellular level. Juices are perfect for spring cleaning the body because they give the digestive system a

> A *healthy alternative to raw fruit and vegetables is to juice them down to a healthy drink.*

rest, help the body rid itself of toxins and their rich nutrient content gives the immune system a wonderful boost.

- Don't go overboard at first. Home-made juice is often stronger than you think. Stick to three 8floz/230ml glasses a day to start with. You can gradually increase this to around six as your body gets used to it.
- Home-made juice should be drunk immediately, because it oxidises rapidly on contact with air, turning sour and losing its vitamin C content.
- Always dilute dark green juices (brocolli, spinach and watercress) and dark red (beetroot) as they are too strong to drink alone.
- As a rule vegetables and fruits don't juice well together and they can give you wind. Apples and carrots, however, are the exception.
- Buy in bulk – it's cheaper and you'll never run out of juice.
- The riper the fruit, the more vitamins and minerals it will contain. Avoid tired or limp-looking fruit and vegetables.
- Juices are best avoided if you suffer from candida, obesity, diabetes, gastritis and bowel disorders because of their high sugar and acid content. It's best to stick to eating whole fruit and it's always advisable to consult your doctor before starting on a detox programme to make sure it won't aggravate your condition.

See p.119 for juice recipes.

> **WASHING LINES**
> Special washes are available that will help remove the chemical fertilisers, waxes, pesticides, herbicides and growth inhibitors that you would otherwise be taking in with the fruit and vegetables. Wash but don't soak the produce if you want to get the full vitamin benefits. You can peel your fruit and vegetables, but remember a lot of the vital nutrients are often found in the skin.

BEST JUICERS

When choosing a juicer make sure that it is simple to use and easy to clean.

Centrifugal juicers These are among the cheaper ranges of juicers but as usual you get what you pay for – they tend to produce less juice per volume of fruit than some other models. Electrically powered, they work by grating fruits and vegetables, then spinning them rapidly to separate the juice from the pulp.

Hydraulic juice presses These produce the most nutritionally complete juices. The press is lowered down on the fruit or vegetable and the juice is filtered out through a fine cloth. They can be manual or electric but the latter is very expensive.

Nose cone juicers These chop or churn the fruit or vegetable as opposed to grating, then force the resulting pulp into a mesh-nosed cone from where the juice is pushed out. These juicers cope better with rinds, stalks and hard vegetables, but they do tend to cost more.

THE WONDERS OF THE SEA

Sea vegetables have long been valued for their health-giving properties and should not be overlooked in your cleansing programme. They contain between ten and twenty times the minerals of land vegetables, in particular iodine, which your body needs for the thyroid gland, the master of your metabolism, to work efficiently. This wealth of minerals also has an alkalising effect on the blood, helping to rid the body of the toxic residues of too rich a diet. Some sea plants

Sea vegetables have long been valued for their health-giving properties

are also rich in a certain type of fibre called alginate, which has the ability to bind with toxins, such as radioactive and metal pollutants, in the body and aid their natural elimination. As our diets become more and more lacking in important minerals and trace elements, all seaweeds from kelp to dulse to the Japanese varieties such as nori and kombu are a healthy addition. Whatever vegetables you buy make sure they come from unpolluted waters.

There are many different types of sea vegetables from which to choose. The best idea is to visit your local oriental or health food shop and buy a few and try them out. The most common are kelp (of which just to confuse matters there are nearly a thousand varieties), wakame and nori. You can either soak them, and add them chopped to salads, or sprinkle them on to your food instead of more traditional seasonings. Nori is perfect for this and is usually sold in packets of ready torn flakes or sheets, which you can crumble.

GRAIN TALK

Whole grains are delicious, nutritious and much easier to digest than their refined counterparts. They are full of natural fibre and a good source of proteins and minerals. They are also lower in calories than many refined foods. A daily serving of these complex carbohydrates will give your body a slow, sustained release of energy and also help to regulate your blood sugar levels. They can be eaten by themselves, as side dishes, or used as a base for delicious salads.

Make sure you only eat complex whole grains such as buckwheat, bulgar wheat, whole wheat grains, couscous, millet, barley and brown rice. These are all high in fibre, protein, calcium, iron, phosphorus and potassium. Quinoa, a small, golden grain similar to millet, is worth including too as it contains twice as much protein as other grains and is an excellent source of essential fatty acids and amino acids. Wheat should be avoided on a detox diet as it can interfere with the absorption of important nutrients such as iron, calcium and magnesium. It also contains gluten which can lead to coeliac disease in people who are allergic to it.

HUMBLE BEANS

Beans can also be included in your new healthy way of eating. They are full of protein, iron and potassium and are a good source of fibre. There are many different types – black beans, lima beans, soya beans, chick peas, lentils – all of which can be sprouted to increase their vitamin content. Sprouting turns a dead food into a live food and can also increase its vitamin content by as much as 700 per cent. As the bean starts to sprout the starch content begins to be broken down to simple sugars, the fats to fatty acids and the proteins to amino acids. The seed has therefore gone through part of the diges-

> *Sprouting turns a dead food into a live food and can also increase its vitamin content by as much as 700 per cent.*

tive process which makes it easier for the body to absorb. With such rewards at stake it must be worth a go. According to health guru Leslie Kenton, the best seeds to start sprouting with are Mung beans, brown lentils, fenugreek seeds, alfalfa seeds and chickpeas.

SPROUTING

You can buy a sprouter from your local healthfood shop but why not do it for yourself. It is remarkably easy and also fun and satisfying. All you need is a large glass jar, some muslin or cheesecloth, and a rubber band. Soak your chosen bean for twelve hours or overnight, then cover with the cloth and secure with a rubber band. Keep in a dark place such as the back of a kitchen cupboard or an airing cupboard if you have one. Rinse and drain your beans at least twice a day, perhaps when you get up and before you go to bed. Within three days they will have grown into delicious crunchy shoots which you can either eat on their own or add to salads.

NOBLE NUTS

Nuts are high in B vitamins, essential fatty acids and minerals. They make ideal snacks to nibble on throughout the day and it goes without saying that they are a hundred times healthier for you than sweets or chocolate. They

Avoid peanuts and salted nuts as they have a very acid action on the digestive system.

are also an excellent protein-packed alternative to high-fat cheese and red meat. Try to buy nuts in their shells as they can go rancid quite quickly. Good ones to look out for include brazil nuts, almonds, hazelnuts and walnuts. Avoid peanuts and salted nuts as they have a very acid action on the digestive system.

MEAT MATTERS

You can include fish and chicken in your detox programme but try to keep it to once a day and remember only organically raised chickens are free from drugs, growth enhancers and preservatives. Deep-sea fish are likely to be more polluted than those from fish farms.

TEA TIME

No detox would be complete without a cup of herbal tea. It is the perfect substitute for your usual cuppa and can be drunk throughout the day in its place. Some like raspberry are nutritional in that they are a good source of vitamins and minerals, while others are better for stimulating the brain and the digestion or overcoming constipation or flatulence.

Beware commercial teas – some contain caffeine so always check the label.

Flatulence Aniseed, parsley, fennel and ginger.
Helps digestion Chamomile, peppermint and fennel.
Pick–me–up Peppermint, lemon verbena and lime blossom.
Stimulates bowels Liquorice.
Vitamin C Raspberry and fennel.
Calcium Dandelion, nettle and chamomile.
Iron Strawberry and nettle.
Insomnia Chamomile, hop, orange blossom and passion flower.

MAKE YOUR OWN

Most herbal teas are now available commercially in sachets but it can be fun to make your own. The best time to collect herbs, especially if you want to dry them, is just as they are coming into

> *The best time to collect herbs, especially if you want to dry them, is just as they are coming into flower.*

flower. Pick clean, unblemished leaves and hang them up as quickly as possible after picking. They should be hung upside down in loose bunches, or spread thinly on a sheet of paper and kept in a warm, well-ventilated room. After two or three weeks you can strip off the leaves and flowers and store them in airtight jars.

Use one teaspoon of dried herbs per cup of boiling water, or three teaspoons if using fresh. Brew in a cup or china pot and keep covered for around five minutes.

WATER

> As your body starts to release toxins into your system you need as much water as you can take to help flush them away.

We are all made up of around seventy percent water and its impact on our health cannot be underestimated. You can exist for forty days without food – although of course it is not a healthy option – but without water you will be in trouble after just twenty-four hours. Water is especially important during a detox programme. As your body starts to release toxins into your system you need as much water as you can take to help flush them away. Also, the more you drink the less severe the potential side effects are likely to be.

We've all been told we should drink at least eight glasses a day and we would do well to heed this advice. Every chemical reaction that takes place in your body relies on water to be successful. It transports nutrients, helps regulate body temperature and is vital to the digestive process and the elimination of toxins. And you shouldn't just rely on thirst to tell you when to drink – by the time you're thirsty you're probably really dehydrated which can lead to any amount of problems including headaches, tiredness, dry mouth and lack of concentration.

If you find eight glasses too much or too little, according to Dr Rajendra Sharma, medical advisor at the Hale Clinic in London, you can work out the minimum amount your body needs by allowing half a pint for every foot of your height. So if you are five foot tall you should aim to drink at least two and a half pints a day. If you find it difficult to drink water, try having a small glass around ten to fifteen minutes before each meal and keep a glass near you throughout the day which you can sip between meals. When driving think about taking a bottle with you in the car.

Work out the minimum amount of water your body needs by allowing half a pint for every foot of your height

HEALTHY HERBS

The medicinal properties of our garden herbs are well known and a few are especially useful in a detox diet. Use them to add taste and texture to wholesome grains and light salads.

Coriander does wonders for the digestion and its seeds are said to stimulate the appetite and relieve colic and flatulence. Use it to flavour salad dressings, or as a substitute for salt.

Parsley is as natural diuretic and can be used to garnish or to add flavour to dishes and it tastes wonderful in salads. It's also good for cleansing the blood and can be chewed to counteract 'garlic breath'.

Rosemary helps to promote good liver function and to stimulate the circulation. Try it chopped over grilled chicken. Rosemary tea can be used as a mouthwash to counteract bad breath which you may experience as you start to detoxify. Simply steep a teaspoon of dried flowering tops or leaves in half a cup of water. Don't drink more than one cup a day.

Thyme can help to relax the digestive tract and is said to work wonders for constipation. It can also be made into a tea by infusing 1-4g of the dried herb in a cup of hot water – you can sweeten it with honey.

Garlic is a natural antibiotic with strong germ-killing powers. Louis Pasteur discovered the power of penicillin in the fight against baceria, but he also noted that garlic juice

> *Garlic is a natural antibiotic with strong germ-killing powers..*

had a similar although less powerful effect. The juice can help to kill off a wide range of common bacteria that cause stomach upsets, including salmonella. It also stimulates all the digestive organs, as well as being an excellent blood cleanser. Although garlic does contain potassium, iron, calcium and vitamins A, B and C, the real secret of its power lies in a substance called allicin, which is produced only when a clove is cut, crushed or heated. Garlic is best eaten raw as it tends to lose some of its strength when cooked. If you can't bear the smell or taste of it on your breath, try chewing a piece of parsley or mint.

TAMARI TRUTHS
Tamari is a type of soya sauce that is made from fermented soy beans which you can use to season your detox meals. It contains no wheat so is preferable to other types of soya sauce, but as it contains sea salt it should still be used in moderation.

OIL AND VINEGAR

Cold-pressed oils During your detox try to stick to fresh, unrefined cold-pressed oils. These are preferable to other oils because they have been extracted from the raw seeds under mechanical pressure, rather than by heat and chemical processes. Cold-pressed oils also contain essential fatty acids in a form which your body can easily use. Olive oil has a good flavour, but if you prefer something lighter, go for sunflower or sesame.

Apple cider vinegar Containing malic acid which helps digestion, this should be your first choice during a detox. Most other vinegars, with the exception of naturally fermented wine vinegar, contain acetic acid. As acetic acid interferes with digestion and absorption of food, they should be avoided.

SEEDS OF GOODNESS

Powerhouses of natural energy and goodness, seeds make excellent snacks and are delicious added to salads or whole grains.

Sesame seeds
These tiny bitter seeds come from one of the oldest cultivated plants and offer a range of healthy benefits. With a twenty-five per cent protein content, they are also rich in vitamins A and E plus most of the B vitamins. They are also a good source of calcium and potassium and contain an in-built antioxidant, sesamin, which has been shown to inhibit cholesterol absorption from food and reduce cholesterol production in the liver. A delicious way of enjoying sesame seeds is as tahini, a smooth sesame paste available from health food stores.Try it spread on bread or use as a topping for grains and potatoes.

Sunflower seeds
High in polyunsaturates, sunflower seeds are a good source of protein and vitamins B and E. According to folklore they have long been used to treat constipation. Due to their concentration of omega 6 fat acids, they also help to protect the heart and are a good brain food. Try sprinkling them on to museli or salads.

Pumpkin seeds
These originate from a specific type of pumpkin grown in Mexico.They are an excellent source of protein, vitamin E and essential fatty acids. Sprinkle them on to breakfast cereals or use them to enrich salads.

BUYING AND STORING

- Buy organic seeds if possible.
- Seeds should be sealed and kept in a cool, dark place.
- Test for freshness by smelling seeds before eating. Throw rancid seeds away.
- Eat seeds little and often rather than in large quantities. They are a highly concentrated food source and because of their high-fat content, could pile on the pounds if eaten to excess.

DETOX EXTRAS

Years of bad eating habits and a digestion system that has slowed down and become sluggish mean that our bodies sometimes find it hard to shift toxins through improved diet alone. A little helping hand doesn't go amiss. There are a number of herbs, superfoods and supplements that can

There are a number of herbs, superfoods and supplements that can greatly aid the process by cleansing and stimulating our organs of elimination, such as the liver and gut.

greatly aid the process by cleansing and stimulating our organs of elimination, such as the liver and gut. These are by no means an integral part of the spring-cleaning programmes that follow, though, and it is much better to detox through diet. If you do decide to give them a go it is best to do so under the supervision of your doctor, a nutritionist or naturopath who can advise you on the correct dosage. Our bodies and our health are so individual that the required amount can vary from person to person. Also, some supplements might not be suitable for you, so always check first. Most are available from your local healthfood store, but if not the staff will be able to tell you how to contact the supplier (see p. 120).

HERBAL REMEDIES

Goldenseal root extract (Hydrastis canadensis)
Widely used among native Americans who introduced this herb to European settlers, it is usually taken for its anti-bacterial qualities. It encourages regular bowel movements and can have a soothing effect on the mucous membranes of the stomach walls if they are at all inflamed.

Milk thistle (Silybum marianum)
Used for hundreds of years for digestive and liver complaints, milk thistle increases secretion and flow of bile. Indeed, its historical use as a liver herb dates back to the first century. Pliny the Elder, a Roman naturalist, tells us that the juice of the plant mixed with honey is excellent for 'carrying off bile'. Today it is still widely taken as a liver tonic and more recently its use has been advocated as a cure for hangovers. It has an antioxidant effect on the liver cells and is also good for regenerating the liver.

Dandelion leaf and root (Taraxacum officinale)
Both the roots and the leaves of the dandelion plant have been used as food and medicine for hundreds of years in Europe, the Middle East, China and India. Such are its healing properties that if it wasn't such a pest to gardeners it would probably be hailed as a miracle herb! It is a good digestive tonic and can be bought as a herbal tea. As a food the dandelion should be eaten as a vegetable – its tender young leaves add a spark to any salad, while the older larger leaves add an interesting flavour to a bowl of mixed greens.

Ginger root (Zingiber officinale)
Ginger has been popular for years in Chinese, Ayurvedic and Western medicine and can be used to flavour foods or drunk as a tea to stimulate the metabolism. Cleansing puts stress on the digestive system and ginger can help to reduce this stress. It is also said to be good for wind, indigestion and nausea.

Yellow dock root (Rumex crispus)

Throughout history, bitter herbs that activate digestive enzymes – such as yellow dock and burdock – have been used to stimulate the appetite and the digestion. They are said to be good liver cleansers and have a gentle laxative action. Both are also said to stimulate the lymph system.

SUPERFOODS

Spirulina

Once the staple food of the Mexican Aztecs, spirulina is a type of blue/green algae that grows in abundance in warm fresh water. It is more than sixty percent protein, making it one of the most nutritious plants on earth and it is rich in essential amino acids, which are so important for digestion. The fact that it contains practically every antioxidant going, including the vitamins A (in the form of beta carotene), C and E makes it an especially valuable detox aid, and as though this is not enough, it is also rich in gamma linolenic acid (GLA) one of the essential fatty acids responsible for rebuilding cell walls – strong cell walls are important for successful elimination of waste.

Chlorophyll

Often used in Chinese medicine to regenerate the liver, chlorophyll has anti-bacterial and anti-inflammatory properties. It is also a mild diuretic and is said to help keep the intestinal flora balance weighed in favour of the friendly bacteria. It can also be taken as an internal deodoriser and as such is good for sufferers of bad breath.

Psyllium husks

The seeds of the plantain, psyllium husks are a form of natural fibre and, according to recent research from the USA, ideal for trapping and removing toxins and sticky mucus from the colon. Taken with water, they form a soft, bulky mass that gently scrubs the intestinal walls as they move through the digestive tract. At the same time they trap toxins and excess cholesterol and flush them out of the body. The husks can also help to protect the intestinal walls, reducing the chance of bacteria and toxins getting through into the bloodstream. Linseeds, which are also rich in fibre and essential fatty acids, are sometimes used to the same effect instead of psyllium husks.

Wheatgrass juice

Made from juicing wheat that has been sprouted to the point where it resembles grass, wheat grass is said to be a wonderful source of life-giving enzymes, chlorophyll and other essential nutrients. It is a good source of minerals, trace minerals, vitamins, enzymes and proteins and is especially rich in selenium, vitamin E and zinc. It is meant to be great for purifying the blood and a good detoxifier as it gets to work directly on the liver helping it to eliminate of all sorts of toxins and stimulating its rejuvenation.

MAKE YOUR OWN WHEATGRASS JUICE

You Will Need:
- Organic wheat grass seeds, usually sold as wheat grain and available from local healthfood stores
- Organic soil, compost or a grow bag with a seaweed base
- Several wide jars
- Hand or electric juicer
- Bin liners
- Planting trays (hard plastic confectioner's trays or tea tray).

Method

1 Wash the wheat grain and soak in filtered water for twelve hours in wide-brimmed jars. Change the water two or three times.

2 Fill the trays with compost, about one to two inches deep. Sprinkle the seed quite densely on to the compost and pat down into the soil.

3 Cover the tray with a bin liner and keep in a warm cupboard until

the seeds have germinated. Water daily but take care not to drown. After about three to four days bring the seeds out into the light.

4 After about seven to ten days your wheat grass will be ready to be harvested. Cut the grass in handfuls, as close to the base as possible. It can be stored in plastic containers in the fridge for up to a week.

5 A good handful of grass should give you about an ounce of juice. Use a hand or electric juicer not a centrifugal type. It should be a deep emerald green, have a bitter sweet liquorice taste and do you the world of good. The recommended intake is between one to four ounces a day.

Aloe vera

Known for centuries as a cure all and almost miracle-working plant, aloe vera has long been used to treat stomach disorders, constipation and many other ailments. Its leaves are filled with a healthy inner gel that contains many vitamins, minerals, enzymes and amino acids and research has shown that the juice of the aloe is particularly good for promoting the growth of good bacteria in the gut. It is therefore especially beneficial when taken after an internal cleansing programme. There are many types available, so make sure you always buy organic and keep it in the fridge after opening.

LIVER DETOX COCKTAIL

Naturopath Jennifer Blondel suggests you try making the following detox cocktail which is especially good for your liver. You should aim to take it once a day for three weeks.

1 tbs aloe vera juice
1 dsp liquid chlorophyll
1 tsp psyllium husks

Add these ingredients to a glass of water, mix together and drink immediately because it tends to set very quickly. It tastes a bit like a foamy mouthwash and should ideally be taken twenty minutes before breakfast.

• Jennifer also advocates walking barefoot on grass whenever possible as it stimulates energy flow to the kidneys.

SUPPLEMENTS

Acidophilus

Concentrated sources of protective and anti-toxic bacteria can be taken as supplements. Lactobacillus acidophilus is probably the one we have all heard and read about, but bifidobacteria is another powerful and friendly bacteria and lactobacillus salivarious is good for cleansing protein-based toxins – as it digests protein waste it is ideal for treating thrush. Balanced intestinal flora is one of the best insurances against toxicity as well as a host of other diseases, which is why these supplements can be very useful during a cleansing programme to ensure that the balance remains stable. They are also often taken alongside or after a course of antibiotics, as it is now known that in fighting infection antibiotics often strip away the good as well as the bad bacteria – a situation which if allowed to develop will result in thrush and possible upset to the smooth working of the digestive process.

Antioxidants

Supplements of beta carotene, vitamins C and E are usually known as antioxidants and can be taken to protect the body from potentially harmful free radicals (see p. 12) which may be generated by lifestyle factors such as excess dietary fats, cigarette smoke, alcohol, pollutants and physical or emotional stress.

CHAPTER 4

Getting Ready To Detox

There is no right or wrong time to spring clean your system but the changing seasons are good starting points – the beginning of spring when salad vegetables and shoots abound and at the start of autumn when there are plenty of fresh grapes and apples, as well as delicious root vegetables. It also helps to get yourself into a positive frame of mind. Detox is not about denial but about renewal. You are about to embark on an enjoyable experience, not several days of penance. Try to see it as taking some time out of your normal routine to give your body a real treat. You are going to put yourself on stop for a while, eating only the simplest of foods that will give your digestive system the chance to clear any blocked channels and to kick-start the body's natural healing processes.

> **There is no right or wrong time to spring clean your system**

The first thing to do is to assess your schedule at home and at work. For a detox to be 100 per cent effective it is essential that you can relax and clear your mind of worries past and present. If you are under a lot of pressure in the office, going though a bad patch in your emotional life, recovering from a bout of illness such as flu, changing jobs or moving house it is better to wait until your life is more stable and calm. Similarly if you are diabetic, pregnant, breast feeding or recovering from alcohol or drug abuse, a detox programme could be counter productive and you should seek medical advice before embarking on it.

If, however, the time feels right, and only you will know, you can start to make a few preparations. The first thing to decide is how long you are going to give yourself and here we are giving you several options – a weekend, seven days or a quick one-day detox which is easy to fit into a busy schedule. It really depends on your personal circumstances and what you want to get out of it. You could start off with the one-day programme, then see how you get on and try the two-day and seven-day programmes at a later date.

Whatever you go for it is important to set the scene and to equip yourself with the necessary tools. Detox is not about diet alone. Body treats such as relaxing massages and pampering baths, gentle exercises to boost you mentally and physically and simple breathing techniques to relax and calm you, all have their part to play.

> *Several options – a weekend, seven days or a quick one-day detox which is easy to fit into a busy schedule*

BEFORE YOU START

So, once you've decided the time is right and you feel prepared you must make sure you have everything to hand. You don't, for example, want to have to make endless trips to the supermarket or the local corner shop because you've forgotten some of the essential ingredients. Nor do you want to be bothered with having to answer the telephone or having to cook meals for family and friends. Make sure you let your family know well in advance that you want some time for yourself and that when you say you want to be alone, you mean alone. Then ask your friends not to call you.

The first few days are likely to be the hardest as your body gets into the swing of the new regime, so it's a good idea to start your programme at the weekend. Whichever programme you choose the first two days will be similar. You will be eating the simplest foods – raw fruits, salads and lightly steamed vegetables – and drinking fruit juices, mineral water and herb teas. You will be sleeping lots and have plenty of time for relaxing, pampering and doing gentle exercise.

PRE-PROGRAMME PLAN

• Read through your chosen programme and make a shopping list of all the essential ingredients. If you can, try to make a special visit to an organic greengrocer. Failing that, most of the larger supermarkets now have an organic counter. Always store fresh produce in a cool, dark, well-ventilated place as this provides the slowest loss of vitamins.

• Think about all the books you have always wanted to read and make sure you buy a copy of two or three of them. As you start to wind down your powers of concentration may not be brilliant so it's a good idea also to stock up on your favourite magazines which are easier to dip in and out of.

• Make sure you have the following essential kitchen items:
  juicer   blender
  sharp cutting knife   bowls
  large saucepan   chopping board
  wok.

• Music can be soothing and relaxing so buy or borrow some of your favourite tapes. There are some amazing relaxation tapes around at the moment. Ask about them at your local music store.

- Make sure your radio and television are in good working order and get some videos in.

- Read through the exercise and beauty plans (see p. 70) and make sure you have got the necessary tools:
  aromatherapy oils   skin brush
  Epsom salts   candles.

- Ask your friends not to phone, or just turn on the answer-phone. It is important that you feel completely stress and worry free. This is your time and you don't want it to be interrupted by demanding family and friends.

- Make sure your immediate environment is toxin free by installing an ioniser. These don't cost very much and you should be able to get one at your local department or hardware store. They can make all the difference to air quality (see p. 7).

- In the run-up days to your detox programme, try to cut down your intake of fatty foods, red meat, dairy products, coffee, alcohol – and if you smoke stub it out. Try to include more fruit and vegetables. This means that when you actually start to detox it will come as less as a shock to your system.

SIDE EFFECTS

As you embark on your detox programme, it is quite normal for you to experience some unpleasant side effects but there is no need for alarm – they are only temporary, a sign that your body is getting geared up to expel all the toxic waste it has been har-bouring in your vital organs for too long. In much the same way as you experience a headache and feelings of nausea after a night of heavy drinking as your body tries to eliminate the excess alcohol, so you will feel similar symptoms as your body starts to eliminate toxins. If you start to feel itchy, have bad breath, watery eyes, feel sweaty, break out in spots, get a

> *In much the same way as you experience a headache and feelings of nausea after a night of heavy drinking as your body tries to eliminate the excess alcohol, so you will feel similar symptoms as your body starts to eliminate toxins.*

metallic taste in your mouth, experience back ache, muscular cramp, go to the loo more often, feel fuzzy, irritable or find it hard to concentrate – don't worry. These are just signs that your toxins are putting up a final stand before they leave your body for ever.

When you suffer from toxin overload your liver tries to unburden itself of some of these harmful substances by storing them in your fat reserves. As you start your detox your body looks to these reserves for energy, and in so doing old toxins tend to creep back into the system. The hangover-like symptoms you are experiencing are merely a result of this underhand activity and they will disappear. They are a healthy reaction and the first positive sign that your body is starting to rid itself of some of the impurities that have been weighing it down for so long. If they persist see your doctor.

You may also feel very tired, so make sure you get plenty of rest and drink lots of water to help speed up the welcome exit of toxins. Don't reach for the aspirin. Draw the curtains and try to go to sleep. Comfort yourself with the fact that you are eating plenty of fruit and vegetables so the toxins should soon be flushed out through your bowel. As you are eating less and devoting a lot of your energy to the main task in hand – detoxing – you may feel colder than usual. Again this is quite normal – just put some more clothes on or turn the heating on.

PRE-DETOX DIET

It is important to ease yourself into a cleansing programme gradually. Although in our heads we know that improving our eating habits for the better makes sense, our body systems tend to react more slowly than our thought processes and they need time to react to more wholesome sources of nourishment.

In the run-up days to your detox, try to cut down your intake of sugar, caffeine (tea, coffee and cola), oils, wheat, alcohol, meat and dairy produce (cheese, milk, butter, or anything that is made with these ingredients). It's much better to eliminate these ingredients from your diet completely, but if you find it impossible you can always do it in stages. For example, stop eating meat four to five days before, the next day take out dairy products and oils and final-ly take out wheat and sugar. If you smoke, now's the time to stub it out forever, or at least give up for the moment. Smoking and detox do not go together.

Smoking and detox do not go together.

So in the week before aim to follow a diet consisting mainly of fruit and steamed vegetables, salads and soups. It will be worth the effort and you will find that when you actually start your cleansing programme it will be much easier and the side effects won't be so severe.

Wake Up
Start the day with a glass of warm water and lemon.

Breakfasts
Eat as much fresh fruit as you like but try to avoid oranges as they are too acidic. Bananas are also not ideal because of their starch content. Make yourself a pot of herbal tea or stick with water and lemon.

Lunches And Suppers
Make yourself a wonderful salad of freshly mixed raw

vegetables. If you prefer, you could steam or stir fry some vegetables. You can also include a baked potato or some brown rice, but try to avoid these on the evening before you start your programme. Dress your salad with a delicious dressing and season your rice with tamari. Make sure you use only cold-pressed olive oil.

During The Day
If you feel hungry snack on grated carrots or apple slices. Continue with herbal tea instead of your usual tea or coffee and don't forget to drink plenty of water.

Going Without
The giving up element can be the hardest part of a detox. Junk food can be very addictive and for some of us once we get the taste for sweet, artificially flavoured foods we just want more and more of them. Endless meals of fruit and vegetables, brown rice, beans and lentils may appear dull and boring in compari-

After just a few days you should certainly start to feel better and, hopefully, this new found-vitality will be enough to dissuade you from going back to bad eating habits.

son. The thought of having to go without bread, red meat, puddings, coffee and wine may be too much even to contemplate. But remember the long-term rewards will far outweigh the deprivation. After just a few days you should certainly start to feel better and, hopefully, this new-found vitality will be enough to dissuade you from going back to bad eating habits. In the long term you can incorporate some of them into your regular diet (see p. 93).

CHAPTER 5

Detox Programmes

THE WEEKEND DETOX

This weekend or two-day detox programme is designed to give your body a gentle rest and cleanse physically and mentally. You will be eating three simple meals a day of fruit and vegetables, raw or slightly steamed. Both fruit and vegetables are rich in fibre, carbohydrates, minerals, vitamins and enzymes and, as we have discussed, the best way to gain the maximum benefits from their nutrients is to eat them raw. If you find raw vegetables hard to tolerate you can cook them slightly – just steam them gently or stir fry them quickly in a small amount of cold-pressed olive oil (see p. 108).

It is also your chance to shut the door on the world, to relax and to spoil and pamper yourself. It's important to get plenty of rest, to indulge in wonderfully relaxing aromatherapy baths and skin brushing, to listen to your favourite tapes, and

> *Your chance to shut the door on the world, to relax and to spoil and pamper yourself*

to catch up on your reading. The more you rest the better the results, as your energy will be put into healing as opposed to other body functions. This is an opportunity to clear your mind of the stresses and strains of everyday living so don't dwell on past anxieties and worries. Go for a gentle walk, try some soothing stretching exercises and practise some relaxation techniques.

Remember to drink lots of water throughout the day, especially after exercising or relaxing in warm baths as both can leave you feeling dehydrated. Water is the best natural detoxifier and will help to prevent any build-up of toxins by binding them with the fibre in the fruit and vegetables before they are eliminated. Try to drink natural mineral water and keep away from tap water as this contains all sorts of chemicals and harmful substances you can well do without. If drinking mineral water, stick to those with a low mineral and nitrate content.

> *Water is the best natural detoxifier*

DAY ONE

Wake Up
This is your day off so don't jump out of bed with the lark. Wake up slowly, think about the day ahead and get yourself into a positive frame of mind. Give your lungs a gentle work-out by doing some breathing exercises. (see p. 18).

Get Up
Drink a glass of water – adding a slice of lemon or a squeeze of lemon juice will give it some flavour and help to neutralise any acids that might be lurking in your system.

Have a refreshing shower and try out some skin brushing moves (see p. 70) to get your lymph on the move. Pick out your comfiest clothes. You will be doing a lot of resting as well as gentle exercise so wear something loose – a track suit is ideal.

Breakfast
Fruit makes a delicious start to the day. It also encourages the liver, which is at its most active first thing in the morning, to get to

work on breaking down the backlog of stored toxins. Pick and choose from your well-stocked fruit bowl. To make breakfast more enticing why not try one

> *If you find it difficult to digest food first thing in the morning drink a couple of glasses of freshly made fruit juice instead*

of the fruit salad combinations (see p. 118) but leave out any nuts. If you find it difficult to digest food first thing in the morning drink a couple of glasses of freshly made fruit juice instead (see p. 119). Juices are easier to digest than whole fruit because the juicing process tends to remove most of the fibre content.

Morning

After breakfast, do a few stretching exercises to warm up and go for a gentle walk in your local park. Keep away from busy streets or places where you could bump into someone you know and possibly be tempted away from your day of relaxation. Take your time, make the most of the fresh air and remember to use your lungs to the full (see p. 81). When you get home have a cup of herb tea or a glass of water and start to relax into the day. Read magazines, start that novel you've been keeping specially, or just sit back and listen to some soothing music.

Lunch

Make yourself a huge bowl of salad. There's no hurry, so you can spend some time thinking about the ingredients and trying out some new combinations (see p. 114). Make a salad dressing out of cold-pressed olive oil and lemon juice.

Afternoon

Try to have a rest after lunch. You may be beginning to feel tired as the detox process starts to work. Stay quiet for as long as you can. If you drop off to sleep so much the better, but if you don't why not try one of the meditative techniques (see p. 90). Don't forget to drink lots of water.

Tea

Make yourself a glass of freshly squeezed fruit juice, or brew up a pot of your favourite herb tea. If you feel peckish have an apple or a handful of mixed pumpkin and sunflower seeds.

Early Evening

In spring and summer this is a wonderful opportunity to go outside and watch the sun going down. Take a gentle stroll, or if you are feeling energetic you could pay a visit to your local swimming pool and do a few relaxing lengths. This can be wonderfully calming but invigorating, and it's good for your lymphatic system as well.

Supper

You should aim to have your last meal of the day before 8 p.m. to give yourself plenty of time to digest it before going to sleep. If you can't face another raw meal, lightly steam some mixed vegetables, seasoning them with a handful of fresh herbs. Alternatively, get out your wok for a quick stir fry. Chop up your chosen vegetables and stir fry them in a tiny amount of cold-pressed olive oil.

Going To Bed

Spend an hour or so after supper relaxing in front of the television, or watch one of your favourite videos. Don't sit glued to the screen for too long, though, as just before bed is the perfect time for a warm, delicious, pampering bath. For the ultimate indulgence, why not turn the bathroom lights down and to get you in the mood, light a few scented candles or even burn a few sticks of sweet smelling incense. Fill the bath with warm water and add whatever fits your mood – some calming essential oils, Epsom salts, or if you are feeling slightly itchy, which is quite normal as you start to detox, some oatmeal (see p. 74). Sink back into the water and revel in the luxury, but don't fall asleep. Allow yourself fifteen to twenty minutes to give the toxins time to come to surface, then get out and wrap yourself up in a warm towel. Resist the temptation to potter and get into bed as soon as you can. Don't forget to drink some water and have a bottle by your bed in case you wake up feeling dehydrated. By now you should be so relaxed that you will slip easily into sleep. If you have any trouble, forget counting sheep, and try some relaxation exercises (see p. 89).

DAY TWO

Wake Up
Again there is no hurry, so try to wake up slowly and do some gentle relaxation exercises (see p. 90).

Get Up
Have your glass of water flavoured with lemon if you like, to get the liver going and then it's off to the shower. Spend five minutes on some more skin brushing to wake up your lymph and have an invigorating shower. Turn the shower to cold just before you finish – this will boost your circulation, tone the muscles and skin and further encourage your lymph.

Breakfast
Pick two or three different pieces of fruit and slice them into a salad, or eat them as they are. Alternatively, pop them in the juicer for a delicious and refreshing start to the day. You may be feeling a bit under the weather and have a nasty taste in your mouth but don't worry, this is quite normal.

Morning
Put on some relaxing music and spend half an hour doing some gentle stretching exercises. Then it's time to venture outside for a walk or, if you've got the energy, a leisurely bike ride. If you don't feel like it, don't push yourself. You may well be feeling tired and slightly weak as the toxins continue to leave your body. If this is the case drink lots of water to help flush them out faster, or lie on your bed or on the sofa and try to get some sleep. These symptoms are quite normal and they will pass.

Lunch
Make yourself a delicious salad using some of the Best Vegetable ingredients (see p. 110).

Afternoon
Make the most of your last few hours to yourself. Try some meditation or give yourself a massage. Alternatively, you could visit your local sauna or steam room. When you come home don't forget to drink plenty of water and try to spend an hour or so before tea just relaxing.

Tea
Make yourself a glass of fruit juice or a cup of herb tea. If you feel hungry have some pumpkin or sunflower seeds, or a piece of fruit.

Evening
Take it easy, you should be feeling better than you did forty-eight hours ago. Think about what you have achieved and how you can incorporate your new healthy ways into your normal everyday life.

Supper
Make yourself bowl of mixed steamed vegetables, or lightly stir fry them in the wok, using herbs or a dash of tamari as seasoning instead of salt and pepper.

After Supper
Relax in front of a video or the television remembering to leave yourself enough time for another luxurious bath (see p. 72).

Bedtime
By now you should be feeling completely relaxed and ready for the week ahead. Sink into bed and promise yourself another relaxing, cleansing weekend in the not too distant future.

POST PROGRAMME

How you finish your two-day detox is just as important as how you embarked on it. You've started the cleansing process, you have taken the first steps to a healthy new you, and it would be a shame to undo all the good you've already done. Don't slip back into your old bad eating habits of too many processed foods washed down with endless cups of coffee or tea. Avoid eating too much for the first few days. Try to stick to fruit and vegetables, drink plenty of water and only drink alcohol in moderation. Bring back other foods into your diet on a gradual basis.

• For more advice on how to incorporate healthy eating into your life on a long-term basis, see p. 93.

THE SEVEN-DAY DETOX

This seven-day detox is designed to give your body a slow, gentle detox. It is based on simple foods which, hopefully, you will be able to incorporate into a normal working life. The first two days are

If you can, start your seven-day plan on a non-working day

the most restrictive and you could experience some adverse side effects (see p. 51) so if you can, start your seven-day plan on a non-working day to make it easier for you to rest if you feel like it. Try to make some time for exercise, relaxing and pampering yourself. Use the weekend detox as a how-to guide to spending your day, but obviously how much free time you have depends on your working schedule.

As for the weekend programme you should spend a run-up week following the Pre-detox Diet (see p. 53) so that the actual cleansing programme doesn't come as too much of a shock to your system. You will then spend two days drinking fruit juice and eating fruit to get the detox process going. Remember, the process is also alkaline forming, which makes it perfect for neutralising any of the acid-forming toxins which could escape into the bloodstream as you start to detox. This lessens the chances of any unpleasant side effects. During the next two days you can add vegetables and whole grain cereals, nuts and seeds to start to build you up. On days six and seven, fish and poultry are reintroduced to bring you back to a normal healthy way of eating, a pattern we hope you will continue to follow in the long term.

DAY ONE

Wake Up
Have a glass of water, flavoured with lemon if you wish.

Breakfast, Lunch, Tea and Supper
Have two glasses of fruit juice of your choice at each meal (see p. 119 for ideas).

During the Day
If you feel thirsty, drink a cup of your favourite herb tea (see p. 36 for ideas). Make sure you also drink plenty of mineral water.

DAY TWO

Follow plan for Day One, but add up to 1lb of grapes and one banana. If you don't feel hungry don't force yourself. Only eat as much as you want.

DAY THREE

Wake Up
A glass of water, flavoured with lemon if you wish.

Breakfast
Two glasses of fruit juice of your choice, plus two or three pieces of fruit.

Mid-morning
Two glasses of water or a cup of herb tea.

Lunch
A bowl of raw vegetables of your choice. The vitamins, minerals and enzymes in the raw vegetables will boost your metabolism and give you a new feeling of vitality. Remember, raw foods are also easier to digest than cooked and therefore help to speed up the cleansing process. If you work in an office you can always take a bag of crudités with you to eat at your desk.

Tea
A cup of your favourite herb tea.

Early Evening
Two glasses of water.

Supper
A bowl of lightly cooked vegetables (either steam or stir fry). Use a combination of three or four vegetables (see p116) and season with tamari.

DAY FOUR

Wake Up
A glass of warm water, flavoured with lemon if you wish.

Breakfast
Two glasses of fruit juice and two or three pieces of fruit.

Mid-morning
Two glasses of water, or a cup of herb tea.

Lunch

A bowl of raw vegetables or a salad sprinkled with pumpkin, sesame and sunflower seeds or blanched almonds. You can also have some boiled short-grain brown rice or buckwheat.

Tea

A cup of your favourite herb tea and a handful of mixed pumpkin and sesame seeds.

Supper

A bowl of steamed or stir-fried vegetables with boiled brown rice.

DAY FIVE

Breakfast

Two glasses of freshly squeezed or pressed fruit juice and two or three pieces of fruit.

Mid-morning

A glass of water or a cup of herb tea

Lunch

4oz of poached or grilled fish and a bowl of raw vegetables sprinkled with pumpkin, sesame and sunflower seeds or some blanched almonds. You can also have some boiled short-grain brown rice or buckwheat.

Tea

A cup of herb tea and a handful of mixed pumpkin and sesame seeds.

Supper

As for Day Four.

DAY SIX AND DAY SEVEN

Breakfast And Lunch
As for Day Five

Supper
4oz of chicken roasted without the skin, or poached. A bowl of mixed vegetables, steamed or stir fried with boiled short-grain brown rice, millet or buckwheat.

POST PROGRAMME

As on the weekend programme, it is advisable to come out of your detox days gradually. This way, you are more likely to stick with your new eating habits and, hopefully, incorporate some of them into your diet on a long-term basis.

An added bonus of following a seven-day detox programme is that it can help you identify any foods you suspect you may be allergic to. Common culprits include wheat, yeast (found in bread, wine and mushrooms), eggs, shellfish, chocolate, coffee, alcohol and many dairy foods. After seven days you should be free of any toxic symptoms and your digestion system should be in good working order. To test yourself for food intolerances all you have to do is to reintroduce the food into your diet and look out for any allergic reactions. As your digestive system is so clean, any intolerance will become obvious (you may feel bloated, nauseous, full of wind, or develop a rash) and you will know to exclude this food in the future.

It may also help to ask the advice of a qualified nutritionist who will probably give you a food intolerance test. Once the offending food, or foods, have been identified, you will be advised to remove them from your diet. The nutritionist may

> *It is advisable to come out of your detox days gradually.*

well put you on a course of herbal remedies or supplements to strengthen your digestive and immune system (see p. 16).

THE ONE DAY DETOX

If your work and home life is such that spending a weekend or seven days on a special eating plan is out of the question, why not try a mono diet – which is basically spending one day eating or drinking as much as you like of one type of fruit or fruit juice. Mono-diets are also ideal after a period of indulgence, for example in the new year after a run of parties, or after a week's gastronomic holiday. They are a wonderful way to cleanse the system and give your immune system a quick boost. According to some naturopaths you can get similar benefits from spending six consecutive Saturdays on a mono-diet as you would from spending a week on a detox plan. Again, to get the maximum benefit from your one-day detox, try to incorporate some skin brushing and gentle exercise, such as relaxation stretches (see p. 86).

It is better to try to stick to one type of fruit so as not to confuse your body with a variety of tastes and textures. This way you will be giving your digestive system the least amount of work. Grapes and melons are popular choices. Whether you go for the whole fruit or the juice is up to you. Juices are certainly easier and faster to digest because much of the fibre will have been removed in the juicing process. Their high water content will help to flush out your digestive tract and your kidneys, and will help to purify your blood in a very short time. Juices also contain about ninety-five percent of the food value of whole fruit

> One-day detoxes are also ideal after a period of indulgence, for example in the new year after a run of parties, or after a week's gastronomic holiday.

and this package of vitamins, enzymes and nutrients are released straight into your bloodstream in just a few minutes.

Like the weekend and the seven-day programmes, the aim of the mono-diet is to give your digestion a rest and to give your system a gentle cleanse. Fruits are great cleansers and revitalisers. They are also a valuable source of vitamins, minerals and amino acids, which are all essential to your general well-being. Remember, as with all detox programmes, to modify your diet for a few days before you start. Try to eat less processed food and fewer dairy products and to cut back on alcohol and cigarettes. Similarly, after your day on fruit, ease yourself gently back into your normal eating habits (see p. 66).

Drink as much as you like of your chosen fruit juice over the day and don't forget to dilute each serving with water. Fruit juices are high in natural sugars and when you drink them alone without food or water they can make you feel faint.

- You should only go on an unsupervised juice detox for 24 hours and you should not even consider it if you are pregnant, breast feeding, severely underweight, diabetic, suffering from a kidney or heart disease, or if you suffer from any type of eating disorder.

CHAPTER 6

Detox Treats

Any detox programme will be greatly enhanced if you include some therapeutic beauty treats. Remember – detox is not just about what you should and shouldn't eat. It is also about destressing and re-energising your life and spending time on soothing massage, relaxing baths and gentle skin brushing will help you to achieve just that. Your skin is also one of the biggest organs of elimination and these treatments will support it in getting rid of toxins. Bathing helps to wash toxins from the surface of your skin and to open up the pores, providing a quick escape route for more to exit through. Skin brushing removes dead cells from the skin and helps to stimulate the lymph, while lymphatic massage has the same effect as well as promoting deep relaxation.

SKIN BRUSHING

This is an invigorating way to start the day and has huge bene-fits. Giving your skin a daily brush unblocks the pores so that it can eliminate uric acid and other poisons quickly and effective-ly, taking some of the strain off your liver and kidneys.

Skin brushing is also a good way to kick-start a sluggish

lymphatic system into action. Waste material is carried away from your cells by the lymph and skin brushing helps to get this waste material moving near the surface of your skin. It also stimulates your sweat glands and increases blood circulation to your vital organs and body tissues.

And there's good news for those of us who possess cellulite-ridden thighs – skin brushing is said to help break down these areas of concentrated excess proteins, fats and waste materials, which are thought to be partly due to a sluggish lymphatic system.

Aim for at least five minutes of skin brushing every day – make it part of your daily getting-up ritual. The first step is to equip yourself with the right tool for the job – a natural bristle body brush with a long or short handle. A long handle is useful for reaching your back, while you can apply more pressure with a short handled brush to areas that are more accessible. The traditional Chinese method used the dried fibres of a gourd – the loofah – but a good quality body brush will do the job just as well.

> *Skin brushing is good news for those of us who possess cellulite-ridden thighs*

The best time to brush is before your bath or shower when your skin is dry. Use long, sweeping strokes and brush all over your body and always towards your heart – up your arms from your hands to your shoulders; up your legs from the tips of your toes, over your knees, up over each thigh to your buttocks. Use circular movements towards the inner thigh where the lymph glands are situated. Then start on your back, brushing upwards as far as you can reach. Finally brush downwards from your neck over your chest and upper back. You can use as much pressure as you want – but go gently to start with. If your skin looks red or feels itchy or irritated, you are brushing too hard. You can start to increase the pressure as your skin becomes used to the new sensation.

When you have finished, have a bath or shower and moisturise all over with a light body oil. Jojoba or aloe vera are ideal.

After just a couple of days you should start to notice a difference in the condition of your skin and also your energy levels first thing in the morning. Your skin will be softer and smoother and you will feel revitalised with plenty of get up and go for the day ahead.

- Avoid skin brushing on areas of your body where the skin is broken or in anyway irritated.

WATER WONDERS

No detox would be complete without some water treatments. They boost your circulation which brings toxins to the surface and help to unblock the pores of the skin, ensuring that the exit route is clear. They also promote deep relaxation – think how good you feel after a long, hot bath.

Epsom Salt Baths
These encourage toxic elimination and perspiration and also help to ease any aches and pains. The salts are mainly magnesium which is good for soothing sore, tired muscles. They also have a drawing effect on skin, encouraging you to sweat, leaching out impurities. To get the most out of Epsom baths try to indulge at least twice a week.

Add 450g/1lb of Epsom salts to a hot bath and soak in it for around twenty minutes. Top up the bath with hot water as necessary so you keep up a good sweat. Get out of the bath and wrap up in a warm towel to keep the heat in, and either relax for a couple of hours or go straight to bed – this is the best option as it allows the process to continue overnight. Remember to drink plenty of water to make up for any lost fluid and smother yourself with a natural body moisturiser first thing in the morning.

Saunas and Steam Baths
These work on the same principle as Epsom baths – encouraging perspiration, which in its turn draws out toxins through the surface of your skin. Low-temperature saunas are often used by the experts to help detoxify people who have had high exposure

to pesticides, solvents, pharmaceutical drugs and petrochemicals. A slow, steady sweat also encourages the release of fat-soluble chemicals from their storage sites in your tissues.

The ideal temperature to aim for is 110-120° F but this may be difficult as most saunas are set at a much higher temperature. You could try going to your health club first thing in the morning

> *If you can't get to a sauna you can achieve the same effect by standing under the shower and alternating the hot and cold settings.*

so you can control the temperature without upsetting anyone who may want it hotter. Try to spend between half an hour and an hour in the sauna about three times a week. After you have finished sweating, spend at least fifteen minutes relaxing, to let your body readjust to the normal temperature of the room before having a shower. Remember to drink some water to replace lost fluid.

If you can't get to a sauna you can achieve the same effect by standing under the shower and alternating the hot and cold settings. Switching the temperature relaxes the muscles, clears the skin and boosts the circulation.

Sitz Baths
Some people swear by sitz baths, which are said to aid detoxification by massaging the internal organs and giving a sluggish lymph system a much needed kick-start.

First run a hot bath and place a large bowl of cold water beside it. Get into the bath, the water should come up to your navel, then hang your your feet over the side of the bath and dip them in the bowl of cold water. Stay like this for three minutes, then reverse the process so you are sitting in the bowl of cold water with your feet over the side of the bath and dipped in the hot water. The effect of hot then cold water on your body gives it a shock, helping to boost the circulation which in its turn helps to flush out toxins. If you find the whole process too much of a balancing act you could try using two baby baths.

Aromatherapy Baths
For a wonderfully relaxing experience, try adding a few drops of an essential oil to your bath. All you have to do is shake six to eight drops of oil into your bath and mix them in. Your body will absorb the oils which will have a therapeutic or invigorating effect depending on your choice.

MATCH ESSENTIAL OILS
TO YOUR SYMPTOMS

Tension Bergamot, camomile, marjoram, neroli, sandalwood and jasmine.
Diarrhoea Marjoram, clary sage and juniper.
Indigestion Bergamot, fennel, lemon and peppermint.
Aches and pains Rosemary, sage and eucalyptus.
Depression Bergamot, geranium, jasmine and neroli.
Insomnia Camomile, jasmine, marjoram and neroli.
Headaches Lavender, marjoram, peppermint and rose.

• If you are pregnant do not use essential oils without first consulting a trained aromatherapist.

Oatmeal Bath
If you experience any rashes or feel itchy as your toxins start to say farewell you could try an oatmeal bath. Oatmeal is extremely calming and soothing on the skin. Get about a pound of oatmeal and tie it up in a piece of gauze. Then hang it under the hot tap while you run your bath. As the water flows through the bag it will carry all the moisturising ingredients with it. Stay in the bath for around twenty minutes then pat, rather than rub, your skin gently dry.

Salt Rub

If you find it difficult to sweat or suffer from poor circulation, try a salt rub. It will help to solve these problems, especially at the beginning of a detox programme when your aim should be to get rid of as many toxins as possible. You can use table salt but sea salt is better. Mix the salt with water or a body oil, such as wheat germ oil, so that the grains stick together, and rub yourself all over with it. Use up-and-down or circular movements and try to create as much friction as you can. Rinse off the salt under a warm shower and massage your body with some more oil. You may sweat profusely when you first try this which is good as sweat carries toxins with it. Remember to drink some water to replace the lost fluid.

MASSAGE

Having a massage is a great way to soothe away stress but there is much more to it than that – it can have a profound effect on your physical health. According to Fiona Harrold,

> *Massage boosts the circulation, lowers blood pressure, aids digestion, relaxes muscles and by stimulating the body's lymphatic system, it speeds up the disposal of toxins from the body.*

author of The Massage Manual, (Headline, 1992), massage boosts the circulation, lowers blood pressure, aids digestion, relaxes muscles and by stimulating the body's lymphatic system, it speeds up the disposal of toxins from the body. There are many different types of massage to choose from – the best thing is to try a few and see which one you like the best. During your detox you can either visit your local salon, or ask a trusted friend to come and give you one. Alternatively, try some of the self-massage techniques below.

Manual Lymph Drainage (MLD)

Lack of exercise and a high level of toxicity can result in a sluggish lymphatic system and a build-up of toxins in the channels. The aim of MLD is to wake up the lymph system and get the toxins moving towards the nodes where the lymph is cleaned before being released back into the bloodstream. It is a gentle technique which involves slowly massaging your lymph channels in the direction of the nodes which are found in your neck, armpits and at the back of your knees. It is advisable to go to a fully trained practitioner for this type of massage but you may like to try the self-help routine below. The moves are similar to those used in skin brushing.

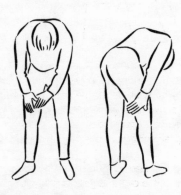

1 Using small, gentle strokes, massage your hands and arms up to your shoulders.
2 Massage your legs up to your groin, using circular movements from the outside of each leg into the groin. Move on to the back of each thigh, again in the direction of the groin.
3 Massage your lower back outwards from the spine to the side of your body and your lower front down towards your groin.
4 Massage your upper body towards your armpit on both sides.
5 Finally, massage your neck, moving from the back to the front.

Head Massage

Massaging around your neck and shoulder areas as well as your brow can often be more effective than taking painkillers for relieving headaches. Try the following soothing moves if your head starts to ache as the detox process gets underway.

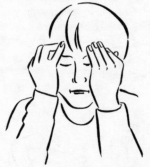

press gently on your brow area

1 Using the tips of your fingers, press down on the muscle running from your shoulder to the bottom of your neck. Use small circular moves and work on both sides of your neck.
2 Press gently on your brow area, starting with the centre of your forehead, drawing your fingertips out towards your hairline.
3 Gently press your fingertips around the under part of your eye sockets from the outer edge towards your nose.

Acupressure

Originating in China, acupressure works on the same principles as acupuncture but uses firm finger massages, as opposed to needles, on pain-relieving points to stimulate the body's own healing powers. It is claimed to help many everyday ailments including digestive problems, headaches, backache, and constipation. It can be practised at home but for best results it is advisable to consult a trained practitioner first. It is not recommended if you are pregnant. The points illustrated overleaf are especially useful if you start to experience constipation, nausea or any sleeping difficulties as you begin to detox.

PRESSURE POINTS

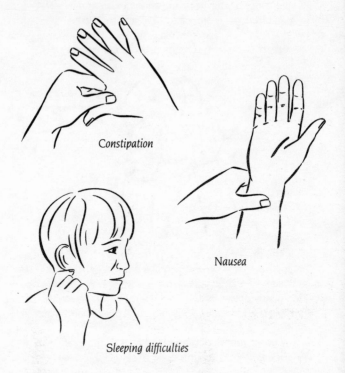

Constipation

Nausea

Sleeping difficulties

1 Depending on your symptoms, press firmly down on the
   point illustrated with the ball of your thumb or the tips of
   your fingers, gradually increasing the pressure.
2 Hold for about twenty seconds, then let go slowly and gently.
3 Wait for a further ten seconds and then repeat the move up
   to five times.
4 When you have mastered the basic technique, try making
   small circular movements in a clockwise direction as you
   apply pressure.

CHAPTER 7

Detox Moves

The value of regular exercise during a detox programme cannot be over-estimated. Your body's natural cleansing and eliminating systems will function more efficiently if you exercise, making you feel much better on both a physical and mental level. One of the best forms of exercise is aerobic exercise, which stimulates your lymphatic system and gets your heart pumping faster, the benefits of which are twofold. More fresh oxygen and nutrients are carried to your cells and the removal of harmful toxins from them is more efficient.

When you exercise you perspire, which helps the elimination of toxins through your skin and you also burn up all over body fat – the body's first storage place for toxins. You will also feel benefits on a mental level. Exercise encourages the production of endorphins, morphine-like substances which help to ease the pain and strain and can make you feel high. What's more, any build-up of the 'fight or flight' hormones that are released during stress can be metabolised more effectively during exercise, so it's a great stress-reliever too.

> *Your body's natural cleansing and eliminating systems will function more efficiently if you exercise*

AEROBIC EXERCISE

To gain the maximum benefit you should go for an aerobic exercise that raises your heart beat to between sixty and seventy per cent of your maximum heart rate (which is 220 beats per minute less your age) and keep it there for at least twenty minutes. So brisk walking, swimming, jogging, cycling and even dancing are all good as long a you do them hard enough and sustain the activity for long enough. You should aim to do them for twenty to thirty minutes around three to five times a week. If you find aerobics too exhausting gentler forms of exercise, such as yoga, teach you how to breathe correctly, which will help you to inhale the maximum amount of oxygen as you breathe in and exhale the maximum amount of toxins as you breathe out.

STRETCHING

Stretching increases the flow of blood to and from the muscles, helping them to flex and relax, which stimulates the lymph. It can also protect you from strains and injuries while exercising and a few simple stretches before and after any aerobic activity are always a good idea. Try the following simple stretches as part of your warm-up before you start to exercise.

Hamstring Stretch
Aim: to stretch the muscles along the back of the thighs.
1 Stand with your feet hip-width apart and step forward with one foot. Bend the back leg and place your hands on your back thigh for support.
2 Keep your chest up and your abdominal muscles pulled in and bend forwards from the hips until you feel the stretch along the back of your thigh.
3 Hold for a count of eight to ten seconds and then repeat with the other leg forward.

Calf stretch
Aim: to stretch upper calf muscles.
1 Stand with your feet together, take one leg behind, keeping

it straight with heel pressed into floor.

2 Bend the front leg and lean forward from the hips. Pull your abdominal muscles in tight until you feel the stretch in the back of your leg below your knee.

3 Hold for a count of eight to ten seconds and then repeat with the other leg behind.

Inner-thigh Stretch
Aim: to stretch muscles along the inner thigh.

1 Stand with feet apart and toes pointing forward.

2 Bend one knee, then slide the other leg away sideways, keeping it straight until you feel the stretch in your inner thigh.

3 Hold for a count of eight, then repeat with the other leg bent.

CYCLING

Healthy and enjoyable, cycling strengthens your heart and lungs, as well as helping you to build up stamina. It's also a non-weight bearing aerobic exercise which doesn't put any strain on your joints. If you live in a city try to keep off busy roads and head for quieter streets, parks or canal paths. The best idea is to get a map and to work out your best route down side streets and alley ways away from the worst traffic. In heavy industrialised areas it is a good idea to wear a mask, available from good cyclist shops.

BRISK WALKING

The great thing about walking is that anyone can do it, anytime, anywhere. It requires no particular skill or training and its health benefits are many. It is an aerobic activity which uses similar muscles to running but with much less impact and therefore less risk of injury. If you do it briskly and regularly enough it can raise your heartbeat to between sixty and seventy-five per cent of its maximum, so provides an ideal work out for your cardiovascular system. It also uses the larger muscles of your body in a repetitive way which helps oxygen and nutrients reach your cells so that they can carry out their essential repair and maintenance work. It is also a great morale booster and if you are feeling stressed or

> If you are feeling stressed or under pressure there is nothing like a walk for lifting the spirits

under pressure there is nothing like a walk for lifting the spirits. How far and fast you go depends on your personal fitness level. If you are not used to regular exercise, start slowly, gradually working up your pace to around four miles an hour. Once you have achieved this you can aim to spend half an hour walking a couple of miles every day, especially during a detox programme. This will give you a gentle aerobic workout, leaving you full of energy and feeling great.

SWIMMING

This is one of the best all-round exercises and you don't have to push yourself that hard to reap the benefits. Whether you are lucky enough to live by the sea or have a local pool nearby, swimming works every muscle in the body, improves stamina and aerobic fitness and it increases your flexibility and mobility. It is also very safe as the water acts as a cushion, absorbing any jarring movements which could lead to injury. If your favourite stroke is breaststroke, try not to keep your head above water as this could strain your neck. To gain the maximum benefit, you should try to swim for around twenty minutes without stopping. Don't forget to warm up and warm down by swimming at a slow pace for the first five minutes and then slow down your pace again for the last few minutes. If you find the monotony of swimming up and down starts to get to you why not try some water marching.

WATER MARCHING

- Stand up straight in the shallow end, keeping your breathing as even as possible. Start to do a high-stepping stride as if marching on the spot. Make sure you keep your balance.
- The resistance from the water means that you can only

perform at slow motion. Use this to your advantage by stretching your arms and legs to the full, pointing your toes and swinging your arms backwards and forwards.

- Sway and swagger as much as you like to produce a good rhythmic walking movement. Carry on for a couple of minutes or until you feel slightly out of breath.

DANCING

Dancing is a great way to improve stamina, strength and suppleness and can give you as thorough a work-out as any of the activities mentioned above. More than anything else it is a great tonic for mind and spirit as it gives you an opportunity to express your emotions and to release pent-up frustration. If years of aerobic classes, step and routine gym work are starting to pall there are endless dance classes from which to choose including, salsa, line dancing, jazz and even belly dancing. When all else fails you can always put on your favourite record or tape and do your work-out at home.

HOW DO YOU RATE AEROBICALLY?

Check out the following exercise guidelines to make sure you are pushing yourself hard enough.

- Your heart should be beating faster than usual but not racing, your breathing should be deeper and more rapid than usual but not uncontrolled.
- You should feel warmer than usual and slightly sweaty, but not dripping.
- You should feel that you could comfortably continue exercising at the same level without stopping.
- As a general rule if you can talk to someone easily while exercising you are working at the right level.

MIND AND BODY EXERCISES

Walking, cycling and swimming require a certain amount of physical exertion, and are great for your heart, muscles and metabolism, but you may prefer to try these quieter forms of exercise with a meditative element that help to soothe the mind as well as your body. For many of them you will have to go to classes to learn the basic moves but you will then be able to practise them at home

YOGA

Developed around 1500 years ago in India, in its purest form, yoga is a complete way of life. Ancient Hindu texts describe its philosophy as a way of deliverance from all physical or mental suffering by gaining control of oneself on the path to perfect union with the Universal Spirit. In the West this philosophy has been adapted and we use it mainly for its breathing and posture techniques, and for deep relaxation.

Hatha yoga is the form usually taught in this country. It includes a number of asanas, or poses, which are meant to help concentration and meditation by quietening the body and nervous sys-

> *This in turn can help stress-related health problems such as digestive complaints and respiratory conditions.*

tem. As well as being an excellent muscle toner that balances all parts of the body, it also leads to deep relaxation. This in turn can help stress-related health problems such as digestive complaints and respiratory conditions.

Many yoga positions include stretching the muscles, which helps to take blood deep into the tissues to oxygenate the muscles which encourages the removal of toxins. During each stretch you are encouraged to take long deep breaths – a useful technique as once learnt you will be eliminating the toxins the body should be removing through breathing more effectively.

As with any specialist form of exercise, it is always advisable to start off by going to a class so that you learn to practise it safely and avoid any risk of injury. Once you've learnt the basics you could try some of these simple poses which are said to be great for gastrointestinal health. Yoga is best practised in peace and quiet so is an ideal form of relaxation for a weekend cleansing programme.

Pelvic Pose (Vajrasana)

1 Kneel with your knees together. Keep your heels together and your feet flat so that your hips are evenly supported by your feet.
2 Slowly sit back on your legs, until your weight is directly above your ankles. Place the palms of your hands on your knee and breathe normally. Hold for thirty seconds then relax, lean forward and repeat.
• This exercise helps to relieve wind and if done soon after eating can help digestion.

Cobra Pose (Bhujangasana)

1 Lie on your front with your hands at each side of your chest, palms down, keeping your elbows close to your body as if you were about to do a push-up.
2 Slowly lift your chest and shoulders, look up and to the side, then come down again slowly. Hold the pose for ten seconds and breathe through your nose. Repeat three to six times.
• This exercise helps to relieve constipation and wind. It is also good for your back and spine.

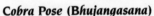

Stomach Lift (Uddhiyana Bandha)

1 With your feet slightly more than shoulder-width apart, bend forward and put your hands on your knees.
2 Draw in your stomach muscles to form a hollow and breathe out, completely emptying your lungs. Try not to breathe in as you pull in your stomach muscles.

3 Relax your muscles and inhale slowly. Repeat three to seven times.
• This exercise is good for constipation and indigestion.

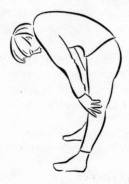

T'AI CHI

Closely linked to the ancient Chinese philosophy of Taoism, T'ai Chi is based on the belief that to be fit and healthy the flow of emotional and physical energy must be balanced within the body. The basic movements are supposed to imitate animals and are linked together into a sequence called the form. This is really a moving form of meditation in which you flow with the direction of energy. It is great for building up strength, co-ordination, relaxation, flexibility, balance and is said to help with most stress-related problems. Indeed, conventional medical examinations of T'ai Chi students in China have proved that it has beneficial effects similar to those of western aerobic exercises but without the stresses and strains. You will need an experienced teacher to teach you T'ai Chi, but classes are available in most areas.

CHI KUNG

Like T'ai Chi, Chi Kung, or Qi Gung, is an ancient oriental exercise which puts great emphasis on learning how to feel and move energy within your body. Some of the basic drills involve nothing more than standing still for anything from minutes to hours at a time just sensing the movement of energy in the body. Other exercises involve gentle rhythmic swinging or stretching movements to conserve and generate energy. It is one of the most successful of all oriental methods for combating stress and is also said to be great for boosting your sex life. As with T'ai Chi you will need to find a local experienced teacher to show you the basic moves. After that you can practise them at home.

MIND EXERCISES

No detox would be complete without clearing your mind of everyday stresses and strains. Your mind and your body are intricately linked and the state of one affects the state of the other. Stressful situations and prolonged periods of anxiety can make your digestive system go haywire and interrupt the smooth functioning of your immune system. Try some of the following relaxation techniques to bring you increased peace of mind.

VISUALISATION

This involves stimulating the body's own healing powers by conjuring up in your mind images of happy places or events. This technique has proved very effective in stimulating the immune system and helping with illnesses such as cancer.

> This technique has proved very effective in stimulating the immune system and helping with illnesses such as cancer.

It often has a marked effect on slowing down the progress of the disease within the body as it seems to boost the immune system and stimulate the production of helpful T-cells. On an everyday level it is particularly good for combating stress.

Learning to visualise a pleasant, relaxing place or event and fixing it in your mind so that you can recall it when you need time out from a stressful situation is a useful technique. The following is a very simple exercise which you might like to try. How long you do it is less important than how often. Doing it for a few moments every day is far more beneficial than doing it for an hour once a week.

- Make sure you have got plenty of time and sit in your most comfortable chair.
- Remember a place you really enjoyed being in. Close your eyes, take a few deep breaths and picture yourself sitting there, savouring the beauty.
- Let your mind walk around, enjoy the sounds, the colours, the smell of the flowers and the shadows of the trees.
- Try repeating some positive affirmations to yourself to increase the feeling of calm and peace. For example:
  ' I feel warm and relaxed.'
  'I am content with myself.'
  'This scene makes me feel good.'
- When you feel ready, bring yourself back to reality and enjoy a gentle stretch.

AUTOGENICS

This form of meditation is a great stress reliever. It involves simple mental exercises and focusing on key words designed to switch off the body's stress 'fight or flight' system, therefore enabling you to deal with everyday pressures.

With both eyes closed you repeat a set of six simple mental exercises which trigger feelings of heaviness, warmth and relaxation. As a result your mind slips into a relaxed yet aware state similar to that achieved in meditation. Autogenics is usually taught in a series of eight weekly lessons but you do need to practise it about four times a day while you are learning. Once you have mastered the technique, though, you have got it for life. The simple exercise below which is done lying down or sitting in a chair is an example of what to expect in a class.

Each of the phrases is repeated slowly and quietly until you feel really relaxed. You then move on to the next one.

- 'My arms and my legs are heavy and warm.'
- 'My heartbeat is calm and regular.'
- 'It breathes me.'
- 'My solar plexus is warm.'
- 'My forehead is cool and clear.'
- 'My neck and my shoulders are heavy.'
- 'I am at peace.'

MEDITATION

Just simply staying still in a quiet environment, regulating your breathing, relaxing your body and focusing on an object (mantra) will put your mind into a state of relaxed concentration. While meditating your breathing, heart and pulse rates slow right down and your brain starts to produce long alpha waves that show you are relaxing deeply. Different systems of meditation appeal and work for different people and you need to experiment and find the one that suits you best. Learning to meditate is a bit like learning to swim. You can to do it on your own but your style and technique will be much better if you learn it from someone else.

RELAX, RELAX

The following exercise is great for relieving general stress and anxiety.

1 Lie on the floor in a quiet room. Close your eyes and breathe gently. Tighten your face muscles for about five seconds then let them go.
2 Gently lift your head off the floor and let it fall back. Keep your neck and jaw as relaxed as possible.
3 With your legs straight, press your shoulders against the floor for about ten seconds and then relax again.
4 Lift your bottom and buttocks off the floor, relax, then bring them down.
5 Keeping your heels together, strech out your legs and toes, then relax.

CHAPTER 8

Spring Clean For Life

Your detox may be over but this doesn't mean you can return to your old habits. Detoxing is just the beginning. Now's the time to work out how you are going to develop a healthy lifestyle for life. You've had a taste of it, so you know how good is to feel clean inside and out and how much better equipped you are to deal with the things life throws at you. This new feeling of vitality is easy to maintain as long as you continue to eat a good diet, exercise regularly and avoid slipping back into bad habits such as smoking and drinking to excess. These goals will be much easier to achieve if you manage to destress your mind. So get going and follow our five-point plan for a healthy new you for life. It will mean making changes, but they can be gradual, and you'll hardly notice them if you go about it in the right way. In any case, it won't be long before you feel and look so much better that you'll wonder how you ever coped before.

> *Follow our five-point plan for a healthy new you*

1 EAT RIGHT

If you want to go on feeling well and vibrant, quick fast foods that give an instant boost are not the answer. Instead, go for foods that provide a steady source of energy throughout the day. These include fresh fruit and vegetables, whole grain cereals plus a small amount of animal protein in the form of chicken or fish.

To make shopping and planning your meals easier try to include some foods from each of the main food groups below at least once a day and follow the dietary guidelines for what and what not to include in your diet. Remember these are guidelines not rigid rules. You can adapt them to suit your own individual needs.

MAIN FOOD GROUPS

Starchy carbohydrate foods Bread, potatoes, pasta, rice, breakfast cereals, noodles, whole grains.
Dairy products Milk, cheese and yoghurt.
Meat and protein alternatives Poultry, fish, cheese, eggs, pulses, nuts and meat alternatives such as tofu and textured vegetable protein (TVP).
Fruit and vegetables Aim for at least five servings a day – three of vegetables and two of fruit.

FOOD FACTS FOR A HEALTHY DIET

Milk
Go for low-fat or skimmed milk – both contain all the valuable nutrients of milk – like protein, calcium and riboflavin. In fact a pint of skimmed milk is more nutritious than a pint of full fat milk because the fat on top is replaced by skimmed milk which is full of nutrients.

Powdered milk
Beware the so-called 'filled milks' which are in fact skimmed milk with added vegetable fat. They are made with saturated fat and

are no better than full-fat milk. Skimmed powdered milks are clearly labelled and are OK.

Coffee whiteners
You may think coffee whiteners are better for you than cream or milk but this is not always so. These products are usually made largely from saturated vegetable fat and often contain more fat than the milk they are replacing.

Butter
High in saturated fat, butter should be eaten in moderation. Try spreading it more thinly and avoid it when you can, especially in cooking. Use low-fat plain yoghurt or cottage cheese in baked potatoes.

Margarines
These have the same amount of fat as butter and contain the same amount of calories. The type of fat varies according to the ingredients and how the margarine is made. They can contain vegetable oil, animal fat and fish oil, and there is a brand made up of a combination of just about any of these. Even when the process starts with unsaturated oils, hydrogenation, which turns liquid oil into 'stiffer' margarine, makes them more saturated. So a margarine made from 100 per cent pure sunflower oil could end up quite saturated. Look for a label which states that the product is 'Low In Cholesterol' and 'High In Polyunsaturates'.

Cheese
Cheeses range from high to low fat but inadequate labelling sometimes makes it difficult to know which is which. The fat content of our more popular cheeses is as follows:
Low-fat cheese (up to fifteen percent) Cottage, Ricotta, curd cheese and Quark.
Medium-fat cheese (fifteen to twenty-five percent) Brie, Gouda, Camembert and Edam.
High-fat cheese (twenty-five to fifty percent) Cheddar, Cheshire, Gloucester, Parmesan, Dolcelatte, Cambozola, Stilton, cream

cheese, Danish Blue, Roquefort, Gorgonzola and most processed cheese spreads.

- Eat cheese in moderation and high fat cheese only occasionally. Remember that 3oz of Cheddar has almost as much fat as 1oz of butter and is made from saturated fat.

Bread
Use only wholegrain breads, rice cakes, oatcakes and Ryvita which are lower in calories than bread.

Meat
Red meat is high in saturated fat and often injected with growth hormones and antibiotics. Processed meats such as sausages and salami contain large quantities of fat as well as salt, sugar, colouring and many other chemicals and should be avoided as should offal meats such as liver and brains. Eat free-range chicken and fish instead or try meat alternatives such as tofu and textured vegetable protein (TVP).

Eggs
Try to eat no more than three or four a week and then only boiled or poached – never fried. Always eat them cooked – uncooked egg white is hard to digest and prevents the absorption of the B vitamin biotin. Beware of foods such as meringues and mayonnaise that contain uncooked eggs.

Fruits
Fresh fruits are full of minerals and vitamins, natural sugar and fibre and are best eaten raw because many of the fragile nutrients are destroyed by cooking. Nevertheless, they should not be eaten in huge quantities on a daily basis. Ideally, no more than half a dozen pieces of fruit should be eaten each day, and less of those that are especially high in sugar such as grapes, plums and apricots. Dried fruits should be eaten in moderation as they can be bad for your teeth. Being sticky they take a while to chew, allowing bacteria in the mouth to be exposed to sugar for a long time, especially when eaten between meals.

Grains

Most of the calories, carbohydrates, fat, protein and fibre in your diet should come from grains and you should eat a wide variety – whole barley, buckwheat, corn, oats, rice and millet. Brown rice should be a staple in your diet. It's an excellent food, low in fat and rich in vitamins and minerals. Make sure you always eat whole grains and try to include them in some form – as cereal, pasta or bread – in every meal.

Legumes

These are the edible seeds of plants and are contained in pods. Examples include blackeye peas, lentils, lima beans, split peas, kidney beans, chick peas, soya beans, soybean curd (tofu) and white beans. They are a rich source of protein, and are especially high in lysine, the amino acid in which grains tend to be low. They also contain many valuable vitamins and minerals and are an excellent source of fibre.

Nuts and Seeds

These whole natural foods contain many valuable minerals and vitamins but should be eaten in small amounts because of their high oil content. Little amounts of the smaller seeds such as caraway, poppy and sesame can be used in baking, salad dressings and as condiments.

Oils

Never assume that if an oil is labelled vegetable oil it must be good – it isn't. Avoid labels which read blended or mixed as they can contain a lot of saturated fat. Palm and coconut oil, for example, are often included in blended vegetable oils because they are cheap. Always go for specifically named vegetable oils like: safflower, sunflower, maize, sesame, soya and olive. Make sure the oil contains only the named oil.

Breakfast Cereals

Most breakfast cereals are made from refined flours which contain little of the original grain fibre. They are also often high in sugar and salt. It is much better to get bran fibre from unsweetened museli and good old-fashioned porridge oats.

Salt

There is evidence that just as different people are born with varying susceptibility to disease about twenty percent of us may be especially susceptible to salt. The culprit in salt is sodium, which our bodies use to regulate many functions including conduction of nerve impulses, the beating of the heart and the control of fluid volume in the circulatory system. We only need around half a teaspoon a day to fulfil this requirement, but most of us are probably getting through about five times this amount. And since a high intake has been linked to raised blood pressure, which increases the risk of developing heart disease and strokes, you should aim to reduce your salt intake by about a quarter. You must also watch out for the hidden salt in processed foods as well as what you add at the table or in cooking.

Watch out for the hidden salt in processed food

Examples of high-salt food unless marked 'No Added Salt or 'Low Sodium' on the label include:

Cereals All bought breads, cakes and biscuits, breakfast cereals, packet cake-mixes and pastry mixes.

Tinned foods All tinned vegetables unless specially marked, tinned soups, meats and baked beans and tinned fish.

Dairy food Nearly all cheese is high in salt, as are concentrated milk foods like skimmed milk powders and condensed milks.

Meat and fish Smoked and corned meats, cured bacon and hams, cooked sausages and salamis, pies and pasties, smoked and pickled fish, fish cakes and battered fish.

Spreads Peanut butter, fish and meat pastes, yeast extracts, lemon curd, golden syrup and treacle.

Sauces and condiments Stock cubes, packet soups, gravy powders, tomato sauce, barbecue sauce, soya sauce, pickles and all flavoured salts including vegetable salts.

Drinks Soda water, some mineral waters and tomato juice.

Snacks All crisps, salted nuts, pork scratchings, chocolate bars and toffee.

• Remember that the aim is not to remove salt completely from your diet but to reduce it.

Vegetables
All vegetables have a high water content and are therefore low in calories. They also contain generous amounts of a wide variety of nutrients and are a rich source of fibre. Unlike fruit, vegetables contain only small amounts of sugar, so they can be eaten in unlimited qualities – but only if served without fat, butter or oil Tinned vegetables should be eaten as little as possible – they have been heated in the canning process and usually contain added salt and sugar as well as other additives. Frozen vegetables are a better option.

Sugar
White or brown table sugar is a highly concentrated and unnatural food. Despite our love for sugar we have no physiological need for it. Any form of sugar is pure calories and contains few nutrients, so despite the fact it gives you a quick burst of energy it should always be used in moderation. It is better to get your fix from more natural forms, such as honey and maple syrup and since honey is twice as sweet as table sugar you can use less to obtain the same degree of sweetness. Molasses is not a natural product, but is a result of refining sugar cane or beets. It contains all the nutrients that were extracted, plus some extra in concentrated form, but it also needs to be used in moderation.

Caffeine
Many people drink large amounts of coffee unaware that they could be hooked on a drug. Caffeine belongs to the xanthine group of chemicals which stimulate the central nervous system, pancreas, and heart as well as the brain. A cup of coffee gives us an instant lift by mobilising glycogen from the liver and muscles and increasing glucose supplies to the brain but the high is only temporary. After an hour or so blood sugar levels start to drop which our brain interprets as a message for more. Caffeine can also cause rapid and irregular heart beats and can stimulate the secretion of excess acid in the stomach leading to digestive

problems. You should limit your intake of caffine or, better still, cut it out all together. Herb and fruit teas, or dandelion coffee, are a much better option.

Tea

Most tea contains stimulants and tannins as well as caffeine. It is probably not as bad for you as coffee provided you drink it in moderation, weak with lemon or milk. Again herb or fruit teas are a healthier alternative but research does show that tannins in tea may help to protect against heart disease.

Tannins in tea may help to protect against heart disease.

CAFFEINE CONTENT (MG PER CUP)

Espresso	150-200	mg
Filter coffee	110-150	mg
Percolated coffee	64-124	mg
Tea	50-80	mg
Instant coffee	40-108	mg
Decaffeinated coffee	2-5	mg

DID YOU KNOW?

All the energy in your food comes from the sun. Plants use the sun's energy to combine water taken from the soil with carbon dioxide from the air to make carbohydrates. When you eat the plant the sun's energy contained within is released, and this food powers every single cell in your body, from brain cells to immune cells. Eating healthily has the power to:

- Improve your mental clarity and concentration
- Increase your physical performance
- Increase your resistance to infection
- Help you to sleep better
- Protect you from disease
- Extend your lifespan.

2 GIVE UP SMOKING

Smoking and detoxing don't go together so, hopefully, you've kicked the habit for good. But if you've slipped back into old ways and once again succumbed to the power of the deadly weed, remember – every time you inhale a cigarette you are also inhaling a cocktail of harmful toxins. Apart from the obvious damage it causes to your lungs, smoking is also bad for your heart and circulation and makes you more susceptible to a number of diseases including some forms of cancer.

Instead of just thinking about giving up, make a firm action plan to avoid falling into the 'I'll do it next-week' trap.

First choose a day when you're going to stop. Think carefully about when it will be easiest for you – midweek or at the weekend – then use the week before to get yourself into the right frame of mind.

SEVEN-DAY STUB-OUT PLAN

Seven Days To Go
Make sure you are stopping because you want to. Check your own reasons against the ones below, then add yours to them. Keep the list handy for the next couple of weeks so you can refer to it. Giving up smoking will make you:
- Fitter
- Richer
- Able to breathe more easily
- Less likely to have a heart attack
- Less at risk of lung cancer
- Have fresher smelling breathe
- More likely to get pregnant.

> To resist temptation you may have to change your habits.

Six Days To Go
Try to understand your smoking habits. For many people lighting up is linked to certain times of the day and situations. To resist temptation you may have to change your habits. So if you can't have a cup of coffee without having a cigarette, try having

a glass of juice instead. Plan in advance how you will react to being a non-smoker in certain situations. For example on a night out at the pub with friends who smoke, or at work.

Five Days To Go
Tell your family and friends you've decided to stop and give them the date. The more encouragement you get the more successful you are likely to be – so ask for their support and understanding.

Four Days To Go
Work out how you are going to stop thinking about cigarettes during the next few weeks. You'll need to keep your mind and your hands busy. It might be the time to take up a new hobby.

Three Days To Go
Stock up on snacks. When you've given up you may find it helps to chew sugar-free gum, raw vegetables or fruit.

Two Days To Go
Try a relaxation technique (see p. 84). Find about exercise classes in your area or check your local library for books on stress reduction and relaxation.

One Day To Go
Now you're ready to give up forever. Make sure you have no cigarettes around. Before you go to bed, throw away your lighters and put your ashtrays in the cupboard.

Remember that you have done the best thing for your health – you've given up and the good news is that as soon you stop you start to recover.

- Just eight hours after stubbing out your last cigarette, your blood will have half the levels of carbon monoxide and nicotine it had when you were smoking.
- After two or three days the clotting factors in your blood will be back to normal, reducing any risk of thrombosis.

- After a year your risk of having a heart attack will have dropped by around fifty per cent.
- After five to ten years your risk of suffering a smoking-related illness will be virtually the same as that of someone who has never smoked.

3 WATCH YOUR DRINKING

Although alcohol is not allowed in detox programmes, there is nothing wrong with the odd glass of wine. In fact, some research shows that a couple of glasses of red wine can actually help to protect against heart disease by increasing the levels of 'good' cholesterol or HDLs (high density lipoproteins) in the body, which in turn lessens the risk of heart disease. It is also claimed that drinking a few glasses of wine a day acts like aspirin, decreasing the chance of platelets in the blood sticking together, so reducing the blood's clogging capacity. But, remember, if you drink more than two glasses a day the harm far exceeds the potential benefits – as can be seen from the resulting hangover. The typical headache and feeling of nausea on the morning after the night before are a sign that your body has taken in too much alcohol and cannot cope with the chemical waste. Also, if your liver has to work overtime processing the excess alcohol it may not have time to deal with the normal digestive processes. And the long-term results of exposing your body to harmful toxins found in alcohol are acute damage to your liver and kidneys.

Research shows that a couple of glasses of red wine can actually help to protect against heart disease

The message is clear – alcohol is only OK in your new healthy way of life in moderation. Men should stick to twenty-eight units a week, while for women the limit is twenty-one units. You should try to have at least two alcohol-free days every week and to spread your allowance over several days instead of using it all up in one long drinking session. To help you stay within the safe limit, one unit is equal to a single measure of aperitif or spirit, a small glass of wine or sherry, or half a pint of normal strength beer or cider.

4 EXERCISE

Cast your mind back to the important part exercise played in your detox days and how much better you felt after exercising. It would be a shame to throw away all those healthy benefits which don't require that much time or effort to achieve, so try to make regular exercise part of your everyday life. It will keep your heart and blood vessels at peak power, increase your metabolic rate and help you avoid putting on weight (a precursor to many diseases). It also protects against high blood pressure and disturbances in blood sugar such as diabetes. And, as well as keeping you physically fit, exercise can make you feel better psychologically. It can help lift depression, boost self-esteem and give you a greater sense of control over your life.

As well as keeping you physically fit, exercise can make you feel better psychologically

Just half an hour a day of moderate activity is all it takes. Thirty minutes a day of some type of aerobic activity five days a week will keep you fit. This doesn't mean you have to go to the gym every lunch hour. It just means doing something vigorous or finding ways of making ordinary activities more vigorous. For example, doing the housework or digging the garden can be aerobic if you put enough effort into doing them. A word of caution. As with any fitness plan it is important to build up gently. If you have led a fairly sedentary lifestyle, don't go too fast. Start off by doing five minutes a day and increasing this gradually as and when you feel up to it. As you become fitter you'll be able to cope with more so eventually you will have reached your target of thirty minutes a session.

> *Doing the housework or digging the garden can be aerobic if you put enough effort into doing them*

It's important to find an activity that you enjoy because if you're going to stick to it, exercise has got to be fun. And you don't have to stick to one type – try running, swimming, cycling, walking, dancing, or going to the gym. According to the experts, you'll see more benefits if you cross-train – mix activities – than if you just stick, for example, to jogging every day. Frequency is also important. Don't try to fit all your activities into one day. It's much better to do less on each day, but to be active on most days of the week. Try to exercise with a friend – it will keep you motivated and the time should pass faster too. To find out if you're exercising at the right intensity follow our guide (pp. 81, 84).

As well as building some sort of exercise programme into your life, it's worth trying to be more energetic. Just a few simple things like walking up the stairs instead of taking the lift, or walking or cycling to work instead of taking public transport can make you feel a whole lot better. They may require some energy at the beginning, but you will be amazed by how much better you start to feel and how much more energy you, in fact, have. Things like digging the garden, lifting the children and carrying the shopping will become much less of a chore than they used to be.

SAFETY FIRST

If you suffer from heart trouble, high blood pressure, unexplained pain in the chest, dizziness or fainting, a bone or join problem that could become worse by exercise, or if you have any worries at all about becoming more active always consult your GP.

TAKE IT EASY

The key to exercising safely is to take things at a suitable pace:
- Always warm up thoroughly
- Gradually ease your body into any exercise or activity for the first few minutes
- Make sure you increase the length and intensity of your exercise slowly – pain or any stiffness are a sign that you have overdone things – ease off next time
- Warming down is just as important as warming up
- Stretch out your muscles, holding each stretch for about six seconds
- Ease down gradually and stretch, holding each stretch for up to thirty seconds
- Never force your body to stretch further than is comfortable and never bounce back during a stretch.

5 DESTRESS YOUR LIFE

Your digestion tends to mirror your mind. If you are under stress your body will find it hard to digest food properly, no matter how good the food. And this is not the only area of your body that's affected by stress. Medical experts believe that it plays a part in as many as fifty to seventy per cent of all physical illnesses including eczema, acne, psoriasis and other skin conditions, asthma, migraine, depression, alcoholism, anorexia, bulimia, indigestion, impotence, loss of libido, menstrual problems and heart disease.

A certain amount of stress is good for us. There's no doubt that most of us require a certain amount of pressure to keep us going, but if you start to feel overwhelmed rather than challenged, it's time to take action. Long-term stress can lead to physical exhaustion and mental breakdown, so learn to recognise the following warning signs before it's too late:

> *If you start to feel overwhelmed rather than challenged, it's time to take action*

- Trouble getting to sleep and waking up early or in the middle of the night
- Difficulty in concentrating
- Feeling anxious or on edge for no real reason
- Losing your temper and feeling irritable
- Difficulty in making up your mind
- Racing pulse or fast, irregular heart beat
- Dry mouth
- Butterflies in your stomach.

STRESS-MANAGEMENT TECHNIQUES

If you are experiencing any of the symptoms above see it as warning and try to incorporate these techniques into your life:

Try to relax. Continue to practise the relaxation exercises (see p. 84)

Talk it over. Sharing problems can bring instant relief and will help you to feel less alone. It can also make you to see things in a different light and help you to deal with stress in a more constructive way.

Laugh it off. A good laugh can do wonders for your well-being and put things more in perspective.

Exercise it away. Channel stress in a positive direction by taking some gentle exercise. Exercising also activates endorphins, the natural painkillers secreted in the brain which induce happiness.

Control it. Try to be in control of situations rather than allowing them to control you. It will help you to face up to difficulties and cope with pressure in a more constructive way. Go on an assertiveness course or buy a good book on the subject.

Stay calm. Try not to overreact whatever the circumstances. It's better to calm down than to make a drama of the situation.

Think positive. Your own thoughts could be the source of your stress. Banish toxic negative feelings and stop doing yourself down. Remember you are just as capable as the next person and at the end the day it doesn't matter what they think.

Be kind to yourself. If you are feeling the pressure, it's even more important to look after yourself physically and emotionally. Treat yourself, in fact try anything that makes you feel good.

CHAPTER 9

Healthy Recipes

• All recipes serve four to six people and can be used in your detox programme or incorporated into your new healthy lifestyle.

SOUPS

VEGETABLE SOUP
....

2 courgettes
1 large onion
3 sticks of celery
2 carrots
4oz/100g mangetout

2 pts/1.25 litres vegetable stock
2 bay leaves
3 tbs pesto
1oz/25g olive oil spread
Tamari

METHOD

1 Heat up the olive oil spread, peel and chop the vegetables and soften for five minutes.
2 Add the vegetable stock, pesto and bay leaves. Simmer gently for ten to fifteen minutes.
3 Season with Tamari and serve.

WINTER WARMER
....

8oz/250g parsnips
1 cooking apple
1/2 tsp dried sage
  or 4 fresh sage leaves
2 pts/1.25 litres vegetable stock

2 cloves
2 sprigs parsley
1oz/25g olive oil spread

METHOD

1 Peel and chop the parsnips; peel, core and chop the apple. Heat the olive oil spread and add the parsnips and apple to soften.
2 Add the vegetable stock, sage and cloves. Simmer gently for fifteen to twenty minutes.

3 Remove from the heat and take out the sage leaves and cloves. Purée in food processor.
4 Return to pan and heat through gently, taking care not to boil.
5 Season with Tamari, sprinkle with chopped parsley and serve.

ARTICHOKE SOUP

1 lb/500g Jerusalem artichokes
1 medium potato
1/2 onion
1 stick of celery
2 cloves garlic

1/4 tsp thyme
2 pinches nutmeg
2 pts/1.25 litres vegetable stock
1oz/25g olive oil spread
Tamari

METHOD

1 Peel and chop the vegetables. Heat up the olive oil spread, add the onions and soften for a few minutes.
2 Add the chopped artichokes, celery, potato, garlic, thyme and nutmeg, and soften with the onion for a further five minutes.
3 Add the stock and simmer gently for fifteen to twenty minutes.
4 Remove from the heat and purée in a food processor.
5 Return to the pan and heat through gently – make sure it doesn't boil.
6 Season with Tamari and serve.

SALADS

COLESLAW

3oz/75g red cabbage
3oz/75g white cabbage
1 carrot
1/2 green pepper
2 sticks celery
1oz/25g sunflower seeds
1oz/25g raisins

METHOD

1 Shred the cabbage, grate the carrot and chop the pepper and celery.
2 Roast the sunflower seeds and add to the chopped vegetables together with the raisins.
3 Dress with yoghurt dressing (see p. 114).

CELERY, APPLE AND PINENUT SALAD

1 head of celery
4 red apples
1oz/25g pinenuts

METHOD

1 Core, peel and slice the apples. Chop the celery and mix with the apple.
2 Roast the pinenuts and add to the sliced apples and celery.
3 Dress with yoghurt dressing (see p. 114).

GREEN BEAN, MUSHROOM AND
BEANSPROUT SALAD
. . . .

12oz/350g green beans
8oz/250g beansprouts
12oz/350g white mushrooms

METHOD

1 Wash, peel and slice the mushrooms.
2 Boil beans for three to four minutes and leave to cool.
3 Add the beansprouts and beans to the mushrooms and toss
   thoroughly with olive oil and cider vinegar dressing (see p. 114).

BEETROOT SLAW
. . . .

2oz/50g raisins   *For The Dressing*
Juice of half an orange   Juice of $1^1/2$ oranges
8oz/250g raw baby beetroot   1 tsp orange rind
2 tbs chives, finely chopped   1 tbs cold-pressed olive oil
                                    1 clove garlic, crushed

METHOD

1 Soak the raisins in the orange juice for one hour. Grate the
   beetroot finely and mix with the raisins and chives.
2 Mix the ingredients for the dressing and pour over the beetroot. Toss well and serve.

CHICKEN AND AVOCADO SALAD

....

1/2 bunch watercress
1 crisp lettuce heart
1 avocado
3oz/75g flaked almonds
3 boneless chicken breasts, skinned
Chopped parsley
1oz/25g olive oil spread
Olive oil dressing (see p. 114)

METHOD

1 Trim the watercress and wash the lettuce.
2 Peel, stone and slice the avocado.
3 Cut the chicken into thin strips and toss quickly in frying
   pan with the olive oil spread. Alternatively, stir fry in a wok.
3 Mix the lettuce and watercress together and add the warm
   chicken and sliced avocado.
4 Roast the flaked almonds.
5 Add the dressing, sprinkle with roasted almonds and parsley,
   and serve.

RAW VEGETABLE SALAD

....

2 stalks celery
1 green pepper
1/2 cucumber
1 carrot
2 spring onions
3oz/75g white cabbage

3oz/75g red cabbage
1 raw beetroot
1 turnip
1 avocado
1 Iceberg lettuce
Olive oil dressing (See p. 114)

METHOD

1 Slice, chop or grate the vegetables and serve on a bed of
   lettuce leaves.
2 Dribble with the olive oil dressing and serve.

BROWN RICE SALAD

. . . .

8oz/250g brown rice
3 spring onions
1 red pepper
2oz/50g raisins

2oz/50g roasted pumpkin seeds
2 tbs parsley
Olive oil dressing (See p. 114)

METHOD

1   Cook the brown rice for forty to forty-five minutes until
    tender. Rinse, drain and cool.
2   Peel and chop the onions and core, deseed and chop the pepper.
3   Roast the pumpkin seeds.
4   Add the chopped onions, peppers, raisins and roasted
    pumpkin seeds to the rice.
5   Sprinkle with chopped parsley and cover with olive oil dressing.
6   Toss thoroughly and serve.

TABBOULEH

. . . .

8oz/250g flat-leafed parsley
2oz/50g fresh mint
4oz/100g bulgar wheat
Juice of 2 lemons

2 tbs cold-pressed olive oil
8oz/250g spring onions

METHOD

1   Wash the mint and parsley and chop, removing the stems.
2   Soak wheat in water for ten minutes, drain and press to
    remove any excess water.
3   Add juice of one lemon and olive oil and leave to absorb
    for half an hour until tender.
4   Mix together and add the spring onions, mint and parsley.
5   Add the rest of the lemon juice, season to taste and serve.

DRESSINGS

For all the dressings mix the ingredients together in a bowl and store in an airtight container in the fridge.

OLIVE OIL DRESSING

3 tbs cold-pressed olive oil
3 tbs Tamari
2 tbs lemon juice

1 clove garlic, crushed
$1/2$ tsp salt
$1/2$ tsp pepper

YOGHURT DRESSING

10oz/300g live, low-fat natural yoghurt
2 tbs lemon juice
1 clove garlic, crushed
$1/2$ tsp salt
$1/2$ tsp pepper

OLIVE OIL AND CIDER VINEGAR DRESSING

1 tbs apple cider vinegar
1-2 tsp honey
1 clove garlic, crushed
2 tbs cold-pressed olive oil
$1/2$oz/10g fresh mixed herbs

HOT LUNCH OR SUPPER DISHES

CHICKEN STIR FRY

....

1 chicken breast, boned and skinned
1 onion
1 red pepper
8oz/250g mangetout
8oz/250g baby sweet corn
1 tbs cold-pressed olive oil
Tamari

METHOD

1 Cut the chicken into thin strips.
2 Chop the onion, core, de-seed and chop the red pepper.
3 Heat the oil in a wok or frying pan and add the chicken strips. Leave, turning frequently, until cooked through.
4 Remove the chicken and put to one side. Quickly toss the vegetables in the oil and heat through.
5 Return the chicken to the pan for few minutes. Season with Tamari and serve.

JACOB'S CHICKEN

....

2 chicken breasts, boned and skinned
4 spring onions
1/2 tsp cumin
Juice of half a lemon

Bunch of flat-leafed parsley
Bunch of coriander.
2oz/50g olives
2 tbs cold-pressed olive oil
8oz/250g couscous, steamed

METHOD

1 Poach the chicken in 1/2 in of water for about thirty minutes or until cooked through. Slice thinly across the grain.
2 Chop the spring onions, parsley and coriander; chop and pit the olives.
3 Add the olive oil, lemon juice, cumin and olives.
4 Mix with the cooked, sliced chicken and serve with steamed couscous.

OVER-ROASTED VEGETABLES

4 medium courgettes   1 tbs cold-pressed olive oil
4 medium red onions   Fresh thyme
2 medium aubergines   Bunch of parsley
2 tbs pesto   Freshly ground pepper
4 garlic cloves

METHOD

1 Slice the vegetables thinly and arrange in rows on a baking tray.
2 Crush the garlic cloves and mix with the pesto. Season with pepper.
3 Spread the pesto mix evenly over the vegetables and sprinkle with thyme and parsley. Finally dribble with olive oil.
4 Roast for around thirty-five to forty-five minutes at 350° F (180° C).

GARLIC PASTA

8oz/250g whole wheat pasta
2 garlic cloves
2 tbs basil or parsley
2 tbs cold-pressed olive oil

METHOD

1 Peel and crush the garlic; chop the basil or parsley.
2 Cook the pasta for eight to ten minutes
3 Heat the oil and soften the garlic for about three to four minutes. Make sure it doesn't burn.
4 Drain the pasta and cover with the oil and garlic.
5 Garnish with basil or parsley and serve.

GRiDDLED VEGETABLES AND RICE

4 courgettes
1 red pepper
1 yellow pepper
1/2 red onion

1 tbs cold-pressed olive oil
Bunch of flat-leafed parsley
8oz/250g brown rice
Tamari

METHOD

1 Slice the courgettes and peppers lengthways. Peel the onion and chop thinly.
2 Brush the griddle with olive oil and put over the heat.
3 When hot, lay the vegetables on top, season with sea salt and pepper. Turning the vegetables, cook until brown on top – take care not to burn them.
4 Remove from heat and serve with boiled brown rice, seasoned with Tamari and garnished with parsley.

FISHY PASTA

8oz/250g salmon steak
8oz/250g whole-wheat pasta
6oz/200g live natural low-fat yoghurt
Bunch of parsley
Ground black pepper
Juice of half a lemon

METHOD

1 Cover the salmon with lemon juice, black pepper and parsley. Wrap it in tin foil and bake for ten to fifteen minutes at 350°F (180°C).
2 Boil the pasta for eight to ten minutes.
3 Chop up the salmon, add to the yoghurt and mix together gently.
4 Garnish with parsley and serve immediately.

PUDDINGS

ORANGE AND PAPAYA DELIGHT

2 oranges
1 ripe papaya
Fresh mint, chopped

1/4 tsp ground cinnamon
1 tbs orange water

METHOD
1 Peel and segment the oranges.
2 Peel and cut the papaya in half, scoop out the seeds, chop or cube.
3 Put fruit, cinammon and mint in a bowl with the orange water.
4 Cool in fridge for an hour before serving.

MP SALAD

1 mango
1/2 honey dew melon
2 pears

1/2 pineapple
1/4 tsp ground cloves
1/4 tsp ground cinnamon

METHOD
1 Peel the fruit and chop into chunky cubes.
2 Sprinkle with cloves and cinnamon and cool in the fridge for an hour before serving.

WATERMELON WONDER

1 small watermelon
2 tbs honey

Juice of 1/2 a lemon
1oz/25g flaked almonds

METHOD
1 Scoop the flesh out of the watermelon and cut into chunks. Discard all the seeds.
2 Mix the honey and lemon together and pour over the watermelon.
3 Chill in the fridge for an hour, then sprinkle with almonds and serve.

HOW TO ROAST NUTS

Roasting nuts brings out their flavour and also lends texture and crunch to salads and whole grain dishes. Place the nuts on a baking tray and roast in oven pre-heated to 350°F/180°C for ten to fifteen minutes until golden brown. Alternatively, place the nuts under a pre-heated grill and turn regularly until golden brown.

JUICE IT

Each combination should give you around one 8fl oz/230ml glass of juice. Don't forget to dilute the juice with water (see p. 32 for Best Juices)

PAPAYA AND PEACH

1/2 papaya
1/2 peach
2fl oz/50ml still mineral water

APPLE AND GRAPE

1 apple
15 grapes
2fl oz/50 ml still mineral water

MANGO MARVEL

1 pink grapefruit
1 apple
1/2 mango

CARROT AND CELERY

2 sticks celery
2 carrots
1/2 lemon

CARROT AND APPLE

4 carrots
2 apples

ORANGE, GRAPEFRUIT AND LIME

2 oranges
1 grapefruit
1 lime

Useful Addresses

The Institute for Complementary
  Medicine
PO Box 194
London SE16 1QZ
Tel: 0171 237 5165

The British Complementary
  Medicine Association
249 Fosse Road South
Leicester LE3 1AE
Tel: 0116 282 5511

The Institute for Optimum
  Nutrition
Blades Court
Deodar Rd
London SW15 2NU
Tel: 0181 877 9980

Tyringham Clinic
Newport Pagnell
Buckinghamshire
MK16 9ER
Tel: 01908 610 450

Suppliers Of Vitamins And Supplements

Biocare Ltd
Lakeside
180 Lifford Lane
Kings Norton
Birmingham B30 3NT
Tel: 0121 433 3727

Bioforce
Olympic Business Park
Dundonald
Ayrshire KA2 9BE
Tel: 01563 851177

Blackmores
House of Blackmores
37 Rothschild Road
Chiswick
London W4 5HT
Tel: 0181 987 8640

FSC (Food Supplement Company)
FSC Information Centre
The Health & Diet Company
Europa Park
Stonelough Road
Radcliffe
Manchester M26 1GG
Tel: 01204 707 420

Larkhall Green Farm
225 Putney Bridge Road
London SW15 2PY
Tel: 0181 874 1130

Pharma Nord UK
Telford Court
Morpeth
Northumberland NE61 2DB
Tel: 0800 591756

Quest Vitamins Ltd
Solgar Vitamins
Aldbury
Tring
Hertfordshire HP23 5PT
Tel: 01442 890335

FLAG (The Food Labelling Agenda)
PO Box 105
Hampton
Middlesex TW12 3TL